THIS IS HAPPINESS

*How to be Happy with Yourself
– Understanding Happiness and
Empowerment for Women Over 40*

Jane Doe

Dedication

This book is dedicated to women from all walks of life who have reached their midlife and are wondering what has just happened, how did they manage to get to middle age without achieving much of anything, especially not managing to be happy. They are sad, anxious, afraid, and a bit angry, but also curious and excited to get into this second part of their life in which they can do things better, make less mistakes, put up with much less nonsense, and try to find some meaning to it all.

Hopefully, they can use this book as a guide through this big new adventure, and as a reminder that they have what it takes to rediscover their powers and go after at least one dream. I wish them wind in their sails, love in their heart, and the wisdom to discover what it is that makes them happy.

Author Bio

Jane Doe is a freelance writer, environmentalist, grandma, gardener, diver and the keeper of a small zoo. She writes about what she knows about—how to be a woman post her 40th birthday, in the challenging world of discovering new horizons, new powers and new adventures. She writes about health, nutrition, relationships, nature, and how all these subjects are connected to create a good life.

Jane went through several careers, two marriages and six different countries, made lot of mistakes, met some wonderful people along the way and discovered that the key to happiness is to open her eyes, heart, and soul to the world around her. That happiness becomes a part of you when you are not looking for it and when you are not motivated by material things and outside trappings of success and prestige.

Table of Contents

Chapter 1

Introduction

It is six in the morning. You have just opened your eyes and you already feel tired. You don't feel like getting up and facing another day of drudgery, just the same as yesterday and the day before yesterday.

You don't feel like waking up the kids, making their breakfast, listening to their bickering before you've even had your first cup of coffee. You have to drive them to school, then drive to work to spend eight hours of meaningless paper-pushing that ensures an income that pays the bills.

Then, you have to return home, make dinner and then hope to have enough energy to be attentive to your husband before you fall asleep exhausted. All you keep thinking is 'Is this all there is to life?"

You might be recently divorced, with kids to raise alone, and in a questionable financial situation. Or you are a career woman who opted for building her business instead of getting married and raising kids.

Whatever path you have taken to this point, your life might look very different on the surface, but you have one common thing: you've just entered the second part of your life, this post-40 phase everyone calls "the gateway to old age," wondering why you feel so powerless and why happiness eluded you.

Dalai Lama believes that happiness is our ultimate goal in life. Then how is it that nobody is teaching us how to be happy? There are no classes in school and no courses at university. We are taught to be productive and successful and to actively contribute to society. Being happy does not seem to be a prerequisite.

And so it starts

After your 40th birthday has come and gone, you started feeling the anticipated changes: getting thicker in the middle despite retaining the same diet and lifestyle; not having as much energy as before; having random pains and aches, worrying about breast cancer and such. Your ever-present anxiety has ramped up but now, instead of worrying about the kids, you worry about your aging parents and whether you will have enough money for your old age.

And in the middle of all that, deep down, you feel like you are not quite done with life. You are not ready to accept that you have done all you could with your career, with your relationships, or most importantly, with your dreams. You feel like a ballet dancer who spent 40 years practicing and now is the time for that dance. All your dreams are still with you. You know how much potential you still have within you that you did not have a chance to fulfill. But how?

This is what this book is about. This is meant to be your guide to showing you the path to fulfilling your potential, getting control of your life and learning how to be happy.

Do I have some secret recipe for happiness? What do I know that you do not? What makes me an expert you should follow?

Ask a happy person

When your car breaks down, you take it to a mechanic. When you get sick, you see a doctor. When you want to become happier, you listen to a happy person. My 40th birthday passed some time ago. Since then, I spent years researching the secret of other happy people, learning what they learned in order to lead happy, fulfilled lives. I read their stories, followed their path and their advice, got rid of a lot of bad habits, and acquired many new, better ones. I learned what happiness is and what it is not.

The most important thing I learned and that I am going to share with you is that you have all you need to be happy right within you. That the deepest secret to happiness is to really, truly want to be happy. And that the change required starts and ends with you.

It is true that after turning 40, you enter into a stage of life that comes with some big changes. Some changes are natural and affect our bodies. Others are the changes that you need to decide to make if you want a more fulfilled life than you had before.

The changes, if you decide that you have the courage and determination to go through them, are life-altering. They will challenge many of your pre-conceptions. They will challenge many things you believe about yourself. They will open your eyes to the best you can ever be. And will chart the path towards the life you dreamed about but were not sure was possible.

Most of the changes will be within you and about your beliefs about what you can and cannot do and about who you are. Not what others tell you and believe you are. Not even what you think you are. You are so much more, but to see that, you need to be open for change with your eyes, mind, and heart.

The toolbox

As you go through the chapters that teach you the techniques, tools, and ideas that will show you how to be happier, you will often wonder: but I know all this. Why didn't I think of doing it myself?

Getting rid of fears, controlling emotions, building your self-esteem, getting connected with nature, all those things are common sense. You can guess that they are something that should make your life better. But you never had the time to do any of them. You had more important things to do. More important than living a fulfilled life? More important than being happy?

We are not isolated islands. We live in a society with its rules, customs, culture, and expectations. You have probably already concluded that something has gone wrong with all that.

Somewhere along the way we have lost the perspective, the sense of what really matters. While busy accumulating wealth, endlessly shopping and trying to stay ahead of the neighbors, we forgot how meaningless all those things are. All it takes is one Covid pandemic for us to realize that. Among so much death and suffering, people were showing incredible feats of generosity and empathy. Suddenly, faced with brutal honesty with the fact that life is fragile and short, we realized what really matters.

Everyone on earth is trying to be happy. Every year, scientists put together a world report on happiness. They actually rank countries by the happiness their citizens claim to enjoy. The United Nations proclaimed March 20th as International Happiness Day. While we know that happiness means different things to different people and different cultures, it is interesting to see who considers him or herself the happiest. Check the report if you are curious.

So, are you ready to embark on the biggest adventure of your life? Are you brave enough to learn all about yourself and all you can be? Are you ready to try things that will be out of your comfort zone? Yes? Let's go then.

When you finish this book, you will be ready for a new beginning. Whatever happened during the first 40 years of your life, this next stage will be better and easier. After all, you are not starting from scratch. You went through a lot. You have scars, stretch marks, and skin spots to show for it. And now you have this guidebook to show you how to build on that experience and make something better.

Chapter 2

Realizing that you matter - the start of the journey

Welcome to the big adventure! You have decided to take things into your own hands and get your dreams back. Did you dust off your supergirl cape?

We have to stop you right here and give this whole idea that you have to be a superwoman a good look. We did it to ourselves, under slight pressure from society. Everyone, including ourselves, expects us to be everything to everyone: breadwinners, caretakers, and beauty queens. And if and when you fail in any of these roles, you become depressed and feel unworthy. It is such nonsense.

Nobody can do it. Not even Martha Stuart, although she has a lot to answer for. What you can be is yourself. But who are you? Before you go on with working on making yourself and your life better and happier, you have to examine this important point: your self-image.

Do you know who you really are?

There is a simple but powerful and empowering exercise you should do: Write down how you would describe yourself to someone who does not know you. Write all your good and bad points. Be as honest as you can.

Then take that list to someone who you trust, someone who knows you well and who loves you. Ask them to evaluate all your self-described characteristics and write their own opinion. Let them add to the list.

Are you surprised that their list has more positive points than yours? That so many of your negative points do not exist on their list, or that they are not seen as negative? Take "I am lazy," as an example. Did their comment, "You, lazy? You do more than anyone I know," surprise you?

Stick this list somewhere where you can look at it and remind yourself that you are much better than you believe. You're not a superwoman but you rock, girl.

This brings us to the ego. The ego is something often misunderstood but something that is an important part of who we are and that plays a big role in our lives. You have to understand your ego because you have to shatter the old one before you can build a new one. And that might hurt.

What is ego and what is it doing to you?

The ego is defined as our sense of self. Not good or bad. Just the way we see ourselves. We build it our entire life based on our experiences and how we interpret those experiences. The way other people see us is also part of it and has a strong influence on our ego.

That means that ego is not real. It is of our construct. But everyone has an ego and we need it to identify ourselves.

We construct our ego by identifying ourselves with our ethnicity, the way we look, our religion, our occupation, our marital status, being parents or not, by our political beliefs, and more.

All these things together define who we are and form our egos. We are attached to it because it defines us, and we do not like it being questioned or attacked. That is the reason for heated debates over religion, politics, or our baseball team. Our ego creates strong, powerful beliefs.

Those beliefs create very strong emotions. It is those strong emotions that lead to bullying, wars, discrimination, and segregation.

Can you control your ego?

Many people are not aware of their ego and do not contemplate or question their beliefs. They will fight for those beliefs when all logic shows that those beliefs are wrong. How can anyone believe that dark-skinned people are inferior to white ones just because of the color of their skin?

But once you become aware of your ego, you can start questioning your beliefs and what they are based on. That means that we can control our ego. And that is a very good thing.

That brings us to the reason we are talking about it now. If you lived 15 or 20 years the certain way, with your particular family dynamics, in a small or big town, in a rich or poor country, your lifestyle formed your ego without you becoming aware of it.

If you became a little overweight after having kids, everyone told you it is normal and you became used to being a chubby mom. If your husband needs a hostess for his business parties, you become one and learn how to dress, decorate the house, and make elaborate meals. Is that really you? You do not question it, because it became part of your identity.

You also live in a society where image matters very much. Where outside trappings of wealth define us. You buy a big house because it defines you as a successful person. You buy expensive clothes to show to your friends and neighbors that you can afford them.

Ego and midlife crisis

Now, let's look at what happens when you reach this strange middle age and your life starts shaking from its foundations. Your hormones make you weepy, insecure, volatile, and introspective. Your job bores you, the kids are gone, you barely know your husband and have not had sex with him in a year. Half of your life is gone and what do you have to show for it?

What happens to your ego? It is shattered. You do not know who you are anymore. You are not needed as a mom, your job is done and your kids are independent. Your marriage is on a shaky foundation. Your job is not satisfying but you need it to pay bills. Do you want to continue this life and continue to be the person you have become? Probably not, but what is the alternative? You need to rebuild your ego to be able to identify who you are.

This is very hard. The ego is powerful. What we built through our life so far is all we know about ourselves.

Besides hormonal fluctuations, this gap in our definition of ourselves is a big cause of depression.

So, what do we do? We rebuild ourselves. We pull ourselves up by our bootstraps as your grannies used to say and build a new ego brick by brick.

This is an enormous opportunity. You need to dig deep to rediscover your core values, your inner strength, your best qualities, and the experiences that you can use to build your new self. Not really new, but a better and improved version.

Mid-life crisis

Let's go into more detail about this world-shattering period of your life called mid-life. The big physical and emotional changes make this phase a crisis. Not the kind men suffer from that makes them buy a red Porsche and start wearing leather pants.

Women suffer from the less visible but no less painful kind. They start wondering what it is all about, why they feel so powerless, trapped in the quagmire of mundane chores and unwanted expectations.

Is it possible that their life is half-over before they could even start doing what they really wanted? We already discussed what happens to women's ego during this transition. Let's see what else happens.

Liselotte's story

Liselotte was a real lady. She was a wife, mother, and the perfect hostess for her banker husband; living in a mansion full of priceless antiques, spending her time planning parties, arranging flowers, and attending charity balls.

But nobody knew the real Liselotte. Not even her kids and husband. The one who escaped Sudetten when the Germans started killing Jews, who drove an ambulance in London in the middle of exploding bombs, who went to Canada all alone, despite her parent's wishes.

But she married nice, calm, sweet Tim who needed a lady. So she became one. Until Tim died. In her early 50s, grieving her husband, after burying him and sending their kids back to their schools, Liselotte had to decide what to do with her life.

So, she dug deep and rediscovered the free spirit ready to fly, and used the second part of her life to go after her dreams. Liselotte sold her mansion with all the treasures, bought a small apartment, enrolled in art classes, went skiing, took part in jewelry courses in Mexico, visited exotic tribes in Kenya, became a tennis champion.

Rediscovering your true self

For as long as you remember, your needs came after the needs of your husband and kids. There was no energy left to take care of your needs, so bit by bit, you forgot that you are supposed to have any needs. You also forgot what they tell you on the plane: "Please place the oxygen mask on your face before helping anyone else to place theirs." Because if you do not take care of yourself, how can you be able to help anyone else?

At some point, usually when the kids do not need you so much anymore and your career has stalled, you start thinking about your needs. And wants. And feeling guilty because of having such selfish thoughts. And not having an idea about how one goes about taking care of herself. Let's look at some simple actions you can start with:

Self-care is not a self-indulgence

Staying physically, spiritually, and mentally healthy is not an indulgence. It is a life-saving necessity. You need to find some time, often not more than 15 minutes a day, to devote entirely to yourself.

Take care of your physical body by getting your heart beating faster by walking, jogging, dancing, biking, swimming, mountain climbing, or whatever. Take care of your social needs by meeting your favorite friends. Have a nice meal with them, laugh, gossip, reconnect. Take care of your spiritual needs by meditating, practicing yoga, reconnecting with nature. Get the inner artist out by spending some time painting, sculpting, beading, and designing.

Respect yourself

Pay attention to the language you use when talking or even thinking about yourself. You might use language like, "I am so clumsy," "I am always getting it wrong," or "I am never going to get it." How about this instead: "I will try it if it kills me," or "I might be bad at this, but by Jove, I will keep trying until I make it." Or "I am having so much fun doing this, who cares that I am not really good at it."

Change your story

When the kids grow up and leave the nest, you start feeling like you have no purpose anymore. You do not have soccer matches, school events, and parent meetings to attend. You feel like you've become invisible.

That is the time to realize that you may just be finishing one chapter of your life, and it is time to write the next one. This time, you might completely change your story. As we discussed before, this time you are not starting from scratch, you are bringing all your hard-earned skills with you, so your options are much wider.

Scared of all the options? Dreading failing? Doubting your abilities? We will talk about those things and work on them in further chapters. They are not obstacles, just challenges. And challenges make you grow.

Midlife crisis obstacles and opportunities

Because so many men behave ridiculously when they reach a midlife crisis, the term has generally negative connotations, even when it is used for women. But this is just the way men react to feeling trapped in their lifestyle, afraid that life is passing them by.

Women feel the same but react very differently. There are many aspects of a mid-life crisis that are painful and difficult. Women suffering from midlife crises start being more contemplative and start questioning and reevaluating their lives, opening themselves up to many life-changing opportunities.

What exactly is a midlife crisis?

A midlife crisis is a realization that your life is halfway over. You start feeling that you have already experienced everything you are going to experience, achieved everything you ever will, and you have nothing much to look forward to.

You start wondering who you are, what your purpose on this Earth is, and whether you did anything worthwhile or made any meaningful difference that will outlive you. These existential questions often bring anxiety and depression. You start questioning your life choices and your identity.

For women, mid-life crisis, which most likely affects them in their late 40s and early 50s, is combined with severe hormonal fluctuations.

Signs that you are suffering from a midlife crisis

Your signs of a midlife crisis range from body shape changes, changes in sexual drive and satisfaction—mostly but not entirely caused by your raging hormones— to emotional problems caused by issues such as dissatisfaction in your marriage and career.

Those of us that do go through a crisis may experience different symptoms, but there are some common signs:

1. Depression

Depression in this stage of life is caused by a combination of hormonal changes due to pre-menopause or menopause and the feeling of powerlessness to do anything about the unsatisfactory life. Thoughts about suicide and actual suicides are more common in this age than in any others.

2. Preoccupation with deep existential questions

Reaching midlife makes women question their lifestyle and the choices they have made – husband or partner, career, motherhood, or the decision not to have children.

3. Difficulty sleeping

Sleep problems are common during pre-menopause or menopause, often due to hot flushes. Anxiety and depression can also affect sleep.

4. Apathy

Many women in this stage feel a lack of motivation, poor energy, and apathy. It sometimes escalates into depression.

5. Thinking of making a drastic change

Some women deal with mid-life by contemplating making one or more drastic changes in their lives, from getting a divorce to quitting their job.

6. Obsessing about good old times

Obsessively thinking about the past and youth as the 'good old time' when everything was possible.

7. Trying to look younger

Obsessing about looking younger, thinner, prettier, and more like they used to, sometimes just by wearing clothes too young for them and changing their hairstyle, but sometimes even going for plastic surgery.

8. Feeling overwhelmed

More than in any other period of their lives, women feel overwhelmed, like they have too much on their plate. In part, it is caused by their fluctuating hormones and in part by the apathy and depression due to thinking about what it means to be middle-aged.

9. Emotional short fuse

Normally easy-going women can turn into emotional time bombs during this stage. They go through a roller coaster of emotions that make them burst into tears at any moment, unable to control them.

What makes midlife crisis more likely

Not every woman sees this period of their life as a crisis. Except for suffering the changes that come with aging, many women keep on going with their lives as usual. Whether that is good or bad is another story.

Some stressors make the midlife crisis more likely:

- Changes in their professional position;
- Responsibilities for aging parents;
- Death of a parent;
- Empty nest, i.e., children leaving;
- Feeling that the marriage is failing or is increasingly unsatisfying;
- Unfaithful husband or partner;
- Regretting not having children;
- Divorce or separation;
- Career disconnect or apathy;
- Preoccupation with 'leaving something behind."

Tips for dealing with a midlife crisis

1. Accept it

You will feel better if you just acknowledge that you are in the middle of a midlife crisis. It explains bouts of crying, depression, apathy, anxiety, and contemplating quitting your highly-paid job and moving to an ashram in Tibet. Once you acknowledge it, you can start dealing with it.

2. Assess your life

Be honest with yourself and dig deep: what is it that is bothering you most, what can you not take anymore, and how far are you willing to go to change things? Is it time to get out of that dead marriage? To look for a new job? To dump that soul-sucking toxic friend?

To feel better short term, look for things that work for you; lunch with girlfriends, a yoga session, a walk in the park, or bungee jumping. Or get a dog. Dogs make so many things better.

3. Stop feeling guilty for thinking about yourself

Give yourself permission to think about yourself for once in your life—what is bothering you, what you need to change, and what do you need to do to make those changes? It is not a matter of self-indulgence but of survival.

4. Do something nice for someone else

Do a random act of kindness for someone, a family member, a neighbor, a neglected friend, or a total stranger. It is an instant mood-lifter, even if you do it anonymously. The old saying that it is better to give than receive is very true.

5. Remind yourself about what you have

Being grateful for what you have puts things into perspective. Many of those things are due to the decisions you made at some point. Look for the meaning and reasons behind those choices. It might tell you which one you should not make again.

6. Take care of your health

This is not the time to neglect your health. Menopause is approaching and you should talk to your doctor about what to expect, what is normal, and what is not. If your depression is getting out of hand, look for help. Your primary doctor will recommend a therapist.

Trying to look younger is fine, but not by affecting your health. Eat well, mostly veggies and fruits, preferably organic. Drink a lot of water, and stay away from excess alcohol and drugs, prescribed or otherwise. Get out and get that old heart beating.

7. You are not alone

When you are feeling most sorry for yourself, remember that many other women are going through the same things. Reach out, find them. Talking with them will put many things into perspective. You will feel justified for your feelings, supported and empowered.

8. Think things through

Try to say this three times fast. Think things through. Whatever changes you are contemplating, discuss them with people you trust. You do not have to accept their advice, but you can listen. Make a list of the pros and cons of anything you are thinking of changing. Do your research.

9. Write a list of your strengths and weaknesses

If you are planning big changes, evaluate what you have to work with: what are your strengths, what can you count on, and what are your weaknesses that will sabotage you?

If you are thinking of changing a career, think about your dream job. If not now, you probably will never go for the job you will love doing, even if it pays less and is less prestigious and socially acceptable. There is nothing wrong with an unhappy lawyer becoming a happy gardener.

10. Find your legacy

It is fine wanting to change the world. When we were young, we thought we could. Some of us make it: find the cure for a disease, build magnificent buildings, and become teachers that all kids remember for the rest of their lives. Most of us cannot change the whole world, but we can change the lives of one family, one village, or even one person.

Find out where you fit in, how you can help, and where your help is most needed. Remember, making a difference is the reward in itself. Do not go around talking about it or posting about it on social media. That is called advertising.

11. Keep learning

Midlife is also the time when your brain tends to be less active. Maybe your work is a routine that does not require much thinking. To fire up your brain, you need a challenge. If you are not willing to start a new career, find a new hobby. Learn a new language. Get out of your comfort zone and join a chess club or reading group.

12. Are you living according to your values?

Sometimes we make compromises that force us to neglect our core values. Did you marry a hardcore Republican who forced you to share his politics? Do you live in a mansion neglecting every single belief you have about protecting the environment? Are you still 'just a housewife' when you always wanted to be financially independent?

These are the issues that will plague you most when you start reevaluating your life during this stage. And returning to your core values will probably be the most important and most impactful change you can make. Being your true self is the best you can do for yourself.

13. Refuse to see the crisis when it is actually an opportunity.

Midlife does not have to be a crisis if you can deal with it and turn it into an opportunity. You are now stronger, wiser, and more capable than you were when you were young and when you made all those decisions you are reevaluating now. Embrace the challenge and opportunity this stage of your life offers. It is now or never.

You might doubt yourself, your self-confidence might be severely eroded by years of neglect, your ego is on shaky ground, and your resilience might be worn thin. But if there is willingness, there is a way. All you need is a bit of help. And help you will get in the following chapters. Let the journey continue!

Chapter 3

Defining Happiness

Once you embark on the journey of a meaningful change, of building a richer life and reviving your dreams, you are in fact building yourself towards happiness. But we know that happiness means different things to different people. Or does it? Let's first define happiness and then we will discuss why it is such a desirable goal.

What is happiness?

Happiness is not a tangible, objective fact. It is an emotion, pleasant, positive emotion that can be strong, such as intense joy, or mild such as satisfaction, contentment, a sense of well-being, or a sense that life is good and meaningful. Most commonly, scientists describe it as a subjective sense of well-being.

Scientists love researching happiness. They are humans after all, and are looking for answers just like we are. So happiness is being investigated and researched by scientists all over the world. There are currently 19,139 articles and papers on happiness in academic and other journals, books, and dissertations. And if you expect them to come up with a definition of happiness they agree on, you will be waiting a long time.

The problem with defining happiness is that it means different things to different people. Different cultures and even different people see their happiness as something else. For Americans, happiness is more exuberant, joyful, and pleasant. Asians consider themselves happy when they are at peace, have serenity, and feel balanced.

Ask five of your friends what happiness means for them and you will have a lively debate that requires a lot of good wine and five different answers.

Happiness vs. pleasure

Are happiness and pleasure the same thing? After all, when we feel pleasure, we are happy. Many definitions of happiness equate the two and define happiness as feeling pleasure.

But, scientists belonging to the school of positive psychology remind us of some important distinctions between the two.

Happiness is a much broader, more all-encompassing state—a state of general satisfaction and contentment with our lives, and our situation at the time. So, while it is not a permanent state, it lasts longer and is more stable.

Pleasure, on the other hand, is shorter lasting, more physical, visceral. It is commonly linked to our senses, such as enjoying good food, good company, or having sex. It is often gone very quickly, like a good meal you spent hours cooking and ate in minutes. And let's not go to how short sex can last.

But, pleasure is a vital part of happiness and happiness boosts the sense of pleasure. You can look at it from the opposite side: you can feel pleasure but feel guilty about it and be unhappy, such as when eating an entire container of ice cream or having sex with a married man.

Also, you can be happy because you have helped someone or volunteered at the soup kitchen, but there is no pleasure associated with it. On the contrary, it often includes hard work and an amount of sacrifice.

Happiness vs. meaning

Having a life with meaning is a big part of happiness, but it cannot be confused with happiness. Many species of animals know about pleasure and strive towards it, but only humans look for meaning in their lives.

In contrast to happiness, meaning is a steadier, more comprehensive state, much longer lasting, not as fleeting and easily lost as happiness. It is a sense of purpose that colors our life and makes us feel that we are contributing to more than just our happiness, something bigger than ourselves.

While happiness and meaning feed on each other, there is often a trade-off. Feeling that your life has meaning makes you happier but at times, in order to have meaning in your life, you have to sacrifice happiness. It is most apparent when you look at how we search for happiness or meaning.

- Considering your life hard or easy is linked to happiness but not necessarily to meaning;
- Being healthy adds to your happiness, but does not contribute to meaning;
- Feeling content is linked to happiness, but not to meaning;

- Not having enough money seriously affects your happiness, but not so much meaning;
- Helping others in need contributes to your life's meaning but not necessarily happiness;
- To achieve meaning in your life, you have to do a lot of serious, profound thinking. That seldom leads to happiness;
- When searching for happiness, you are taking, searching for meaning means giving;
- Trying to be wise, generous and creative contribute to your life's meaning, but very rarely to happiness. Often, they are detrimental to happiness.

What can we conclude from this? That your life can be meaningful while you are unhappy, but it is hard to be happy if your life has no meaning.

The prerequisites for happiness

We agreed that different things make different people happy, but there are some generally accepted conditions that are necessary for anyone to be happy:

- Sufficient basic income;
- Having a satisfying job;
- Physical and mental health;
- Good family relationship;
- Rich social life;
- Living according to your own moral values;
- Experiencing positive emotions.

Are you surprised? Just think about it. You cannot possibly be happy if you are struggling to pay bills and put food on the table for your kids. You cannot be happy if your husband is cheating on you or your kids do not talk to you. It is impossible to be happy if your mother has just died or you have been diagnosed with cancer.

This brings us to a big question: can we achieve happiness? Are we in control of how happy we can be?

Unequal opportunities for happiness

You must be sick of reading how happiness is a choice. All you have to do is follow ten steps or do yoga or write a journal and you will be happier. If you are struggling with low income, being marginalized because of your skin color or because of your sexual orientation, is yoga going to help you to be happier?

Whatever the feel-good articles are saying, your life is proof that it is not as simple. There are forces at work that make happiness much less reachable for some people. A political conflict where you live, racism, and economic inequality are just a few factors that are not in your control and affect your chance of being happy.

Even scientists are finally acknowledging what you know: happiness is not always an individual choice; it is also affected by economic, institutional, and historical forces.

What does this mean for our pursuit of happiness? All it means is that we have to combat more than our ego and bad habits. But we will talk much more about that in later chapters.

What are those structural forces we are talking about? Take slavery, for example, it was a powerful structural force that formed a pattern of cultural, social, economic, and personal relationships between Black and White people. And in many countries, this force is still at work.

Throughout history, men were the dominant power in families, governments, the economy and just about everything else. They influenced laws that are at work to this day. They influenced the difference in power between men and women on all levels: in families, at work with unequal salaries, or when seeking a divorce.

The social position of a person is dictated by the family she or he comes from, what school they went to, where they work, what church they belong to and what club.

You do not see these structural forces at work in your everyday life. You are not consciously aware of them. But they do shape our lives and we became aware of them when we tried to do something or go somewhere we believe would make our lives better, and hit a snag.

On the other hand, it is easy to blame outside, structural forces for our lack of happiness and general misfortune. It just leads to feelings of helplessness and passivity. What matters is that we are aware of the forces at work and count on them as powerful obstacles in our quest for happiness.

Being unhappy is not your fault

This is very important to stress. Why? Because you feel guilty if you fail to follow the advice given in popular magazines or on the internet or they just do not work.

But if you are working two jobs to feed the kids or going to school at night after work to get a promotion, or taking care of your sick mother, you really do not have the time to do yoga or write a journal. Unless you realize that 15 minutes of taking care of yourself would likely make you more fit to do all your chores.

We now know that there are different forces at work that are keeping you from being happier. Some are in your control and some are not. Sometimes you feel like all the advice is meant for the privileged few, who can afford to spend time writing in a gratitude journal while you are struggling with the bickering kids or helping them with their homework.

Do not take this wrong: all those activities feel-good articles mention are hugely important in order to make you stronger and more resilient to cope with what life throws at you. They will make you happier to the extent that they will make you feel like you are doing something for yourself. But without solving your basic issues, your happiness is still a long road ahead, mindfulness or not.

Are we supposed to be happy?

It is interesting to learn that our insistence on being happy is historically new. Our grandparents did not expect it while trying to survive the harsh reality of life. If you look at other countries, happiness is not considered a need. Life is about responsibilities and duties. In fact, the word for 'happiness' in many languages is the same as the word for luck. So, is happiness real, something we can control, or is it a product of luck?

Scientists found that in every—really, every—Indo-European language, the word for happiness is the same as the word for luck. In Old Norse and Old English, the word Hap is the root of the word 'happiness," but it also means luck or chance. The Old French word 'heur," the root of

"Bonheur," means good fortune as well as happiness. The German word 'gluck' means both chance and happiness.

Interesting and a fun topic of conversation at the next gathering with your besties, but we are not going to leave our happiness to chance, right?

Why do we insist on happiness?

Some people believe that the pursuit of happiness is self-indulgence, and good only as a by-product of more important things in life, that striving for happiness is useless, and that focusing on other, more important endeavors might bring greater contentment.

Other people believe that happiness is the ultimate goal for humans and that happiness can be achieved and increased intentionally and purposefully.

Whatever theory you prescribe to, we like being happy. It makes us feel good. When we are happy, we can deal better with life's harsh realities.

When you talk to people who consider themselves to be happy, you will find surprising revelations. Happiness can be having good weather if you are a farmer; it can be getting good news from the doctor; it can be even anticipating something good to happen, long before it happens. It surely beats the alternative. It helps to understand that happiness does not last forever.

Happiness and health

It is common to say that there is no happiness without health. Being sick prevents us from being happy. We have also learned that happy people are get sick less often than those who are unhappy. It seems that the relationship between health and happiness is complex and when they exist together, they provide the two most important foundations for a good life. They in many ways influence each other, but which comes first?

Physical benefits of happiness

Happiness is linked to a range of physical health benefits. It lowers blood pressure, decreases the risk of stroke, boosts the immune system, and prolongs life. Feeling happy reduces the risk of injury in both young and old people.

Do happy people live longer?

Happiness is associated with a longer lifespan in many people. Those who report being happy and generally feel a sense of well-being live longer on average than people who consider themselves unhappy.

Can happiness boost your immune system?

Evidence shows that happy people have a stronger immune system and when they do get sick, the symptoms are much milder. For example, in a group of people exposed to a flu virus, those who are more content, balanced and happy rarely suffer symptoms or the symptoms are fairly weak.

Interestingly, if happiness is intentionally boosted in people for a few weeks before they are exposed to a virus, they are more likely to suffer no symptoms or have very mild symptoms.

Why? Scientists are not sure, but one of the most accepted theories is that happy people normally lead healthier lives, eat better, take care of themselves, engage in physical activities and have a rich social life. So, it means that the activities we found to boost happiness are the same as those that boost our immune system and prolong our lives.

Another possible link is that happy people are less stressed or cope with stressful situations better. Stress is known for taking a big toll on our overall health, making us more prone to diseases and infections.

How health influences happiness

It does not require a big brain to conclude that failing health has detrimental effects on our overall happiness. It is not only dealing with pain, fear of death, consuming medication that is often toxic, or staying in a hospital, but also dealing with medical bills and needing the money for medical treatment when the money is needed to feed the kids.

Good health, on the other hand, is one of the main basic prerequisites for happiness. Everything we do to stay healthy such as good nutrition, sufficient exercise and enough sleep also contribute to our happiness.

Does health bring happiness?

Some researchers suggest that when people take good care of themselves, they feel happier. Other researchers found that healthy people simply have a more positive outlook. Or that genetics or personality traits are underlying factors that contribute to both. Scientists have a hard time saying that they do not know.

Why does exercise make you feel happy?

This one is simple and not ambiguous: exercise boosts our body's production of endorphins and enkephalins, two hormones responsible for reducing pain and boosting pleasure. These hormones are also called 'happy hormones,' and the feeling of happiness after a run or other exercise is known as a "runner's high."

In addition, during exercise, our mind is distracted from the endless churning and worrying about problems and concerns that cause stress just by thinking about them, even if they will never come to pass. This is one big reason why going out into nature and spending time with others is so important for happiness.

Are there *happy foods*?

Extensive research shows the direct correlation between our gut and the brain and mental health. Ingredients in some foods can improve the gut flora, the bacteria that promote brain activities. Some beneficial foods are fish, rich in omega-3 fatty acids, and veggies, rich in fiber.

Is it possible to be happy when suffering from a chronic illness?

People suffering from a chronic illness, cancer treatment and even people in palliative care can make every day more meaningful and their pain bearable through mindful meditation and self-compassion. Mindfulness makes them focus on the moment and what their senses tell them about the world around them instead of focusing on their illness and suffering. The best cancer jokes are told by cancer patients waiting on chemotherapy.

The right to be happy

When you think about transforming your life in your midlife, all the things you want to change are ultimately supposed to lead you to a happier life. You want a more fulfilling job, a loving relationship, time to spend in nature, time to devote to art or hobbies, and the company of people you can trust. You want to keep learning, to be able to help others, and to enjoy good health. You want your life to make sense, to have meaning. If we had all of that, we would be happy.

Now, all you have to do is get out of your armchair, turn the TV off, switch off your phone and get on with it. Maybe tomorrow? Let's discuss what it takes to reach all our goals.

Chapter 4

Empowerment through building self-confidence and resilience

So far, we have covered the difficult and earth-shattering stage of mid-life, what it does to women, and how to face it. We discussed happiness as the goal, where pleasure and meaning have to combine to make you happy.

Now we've come to the crucial point: how to get there. How to use our midlife crisis to make the second half better, happier, and more meaningful. It means you have to make yourself strong, confident, and resilient for the battle ahead. Because it is a battle and these are your weapons.

We have discussed ego, the way we perceive ourselves. We now have to shatter that ego because it is based on our previous experiences and on the way others perceive us, forcing us to perceive ourselves the same way. And shattering your ego is a very big deal because you have to make a new one.

We all need a sense of self. You are going to build a new sense of self—new and improved, and strong and empowered, so you can change the things in your life that need changing.

How do you empower yourself for this battle? Not feeling strong enough, brave enough, confident enough, and resilient enough? We will work on all that, but let's start by looking at what we mean by being empowered.

What is an empowered woman?

When you think of an empowered woman, what do you see? A well-dressed beautifully groomed woman who dominates corporate meetings full of men, who walks with her head high and demands respect? Is that what you think an empowered woman is? There is no doubt that a woman like that is empowered, but you do not need to have a Ph.D., perfect grooming and a powerful job to be empowered.

Do you sometimes feel like all the articles you read about empowered women are written for the affluent, privileged, well-educated mostly white women? Empowerment is much more than the appearance of self-confidence. It means true self-confidence to deal with whatever life throws at you.

- An empowered woman is a widow with three kids and a farm, managing to raise kids so that they do not become hooligans and managing her farm so it does not go to the bank.

- It is a divorced woman who was a housewife her whole life, who put her husband through school while she was raising kids and keeping the house beautiful, who is going back to school at night while working a junior job until she gains experience.

- An empowered woman is quitting her job in her 40s when she realized that working as a money broker is destroying her soul, and moving to Costa Rica to run an environmental non-profit.

So, in whatever position you found yourself after your 40th birthday has come and gone, start by evaluating the situation and making a plan. You might be depressed, or you might be angry. Both are normal, but you need to put your feelings aside and evaluate your strengths and weaknesses for the oncoming battle.

Do you lack the self-confidence to deal with all this heavy stuff? After all, you have never stood up for yourself, how do you start now? Are you scared witless to leave all you knew behind and create a new life for yourself? Let's start with how to deal with that fear.

Conquering fear

Fear is our reaction to danger, real or perceived. It is impossible to go through life without fear of something or somebody. But we can deal with our fears by identifying them, learning how to live with them, and in the process conquering them.

What are you really afraid of?

Sort out your experiences and identify your fears. Not all of them are obvious like the fear of spiders. You might be afraid of public speaking but not realize it until you find yourself in a situation where you have to speak in front of an audience. Are you afraid of the dark? Really? At your age? Do you know why?

Once you sorted out all your fears and labeled them, you will have something concrete to work with. For example, where did your fear of the dark come from? Did it start in your childhood? Are you afraid only when you are alone? Did someone lock you in a dark place as a kid?

Learn all you can about your fear

It is important to become familiar with your fear, its causes and its roots. The familiarity will make your fear tangible and explainable. That way, the fear loses its power. And that is something you can work with.

Facing your fear

There is no way around it: to conquer your fear, you have to face it. Jump right into it. Running away from it will only give it more power over you. Once you face what you are afraid of deliberately and consciously, it will lose its power. You will realize that fear is not real. It is just an emotion.

If dark is your fear, start exposing yourself to it slowly and for short periods. Go into a dark room that is familiar to you and just breathe. Think of something pleasant for a few minutes. The next day, do it a bit longer. Continue until it is gone.

You can do this de-sensitization with any fear you suffered from for a long time. Always remind yourself that fear is just an emotion, it exists only in your mind and you can get it out.

Reward yourself

Conquering your fear is not easy but it is very satisfying and empowering. Celebrate conquering each of your fears. Treat yourself, and mark the occasion: you are starting the new phase of your life with one less fear. You will probably not be able to get rid of all your fears. Do you know anyone who is not afraid of their mother-in-law coming unexpectedly and finding their house in a mess?

Might happen?

Most of our fears are perceived dangers and not real threats. But the worst fear is of things we anticipate, especially things we have zero control over. Equally bad is the fear of something we anticipate but is very unlikely to happen.

You are afraid that your colleagues will make fun of you after they hear your presentation? You know that is very unlikely to happen; you prepared it well and you know your stuff. But your insecurity makes you crippled with fear, so you actually sabotage yourself and stumble through the presentation.

Give yourself a pep talk before the presentation. Breathe deeply and tell yourself that you are ready, you are good and there is nothing to fear.

Try New Things

Why not decide to be brave from now on? You can face anything. You are strong and powerful. Even spiders. OK, maybe not spiders. But it is a good idea to occasionally try new things that are completely out of your comfort zone, as a practice of not being afraid. If you are afraid of heights, try a hot air balloon ride. It is scary but it is also exhilarating and fairly safe. You can conquer your fear of speaking in front of an audience by singing karaoke when going out with friends. It might take a few cocktails to get there, but friends will support you.

It is all in your mind

Every time you experience a perceived fear (what is your chance of actually encountering a big hairy spider?) remind yourself that fear is not something concrete and objective. It is an emotion. It exists only in your mind. And you can control what is in your mind. Do not go too far: this works only for perceived fears. There are real bears in the woods, so be careful when hiking in the forest.

How to control your emotions

When dealing with your fears, you realized that emotions are something you can control. But our lives are full of emotions and some of them literally rule our lives. Learning to control them can change your life.

Controlling your emotions does not mean having a poker face and being all stoic when you want to scream. It means stopping yourself from screaming when screaming can be bad for you, damage your reputation, wake up the kids, or scare your boss.

Controlling emotions does not mean suppressing emotions. It just means not letting your emotions force you to say something and act in a way that can hurt you. Punching a bully that was hurting your kid in the face would be really satisfying but will only earn you a day in court.

Emotions are important. We all feel them. They are our reactions to what is happening around us. Even negative emotions are important and can help us grow.

There is an interesting aspect of emotions that you should know that is not commonly acknowledged: your emotional reaction is not the reaction to something that is happening but to your evaluation of what is happening.

What does it mean? Every time you are in a situation that causes you an emotion—anger, fear, sadness, anxiety or whatever—your mind instantly evaluates that situation and reacts in a way that it considers appropriate. It all happens instantly, without your conscious awareness. It means that not everyone will have the same reaction, or the same emotion to the same situation.

Let's look at an example: your family is going skiing. Your husband is thrilled. Your daughter is angry because she does not want to leave her friends. Your son is anxious because he is an inexperienced skier. And you are horrified because the last time you were on skis you broke your arm.

So what do you do? Now that you know that your emotion is triggered by your mind evaluating the situation as dangerous, you can control it. You can go on an easier slope, go slowly or tell yourself that you will be more careful this time and not forget to strap your skis properly.

Do you see where this takes you? You can let your fear rule you and drown in a negative feeling of fear and anxiety, or you can control your fear by evaluating the danger as real or unreal and deciding accordingly.

This is possible only once you accept that emotions are created by your mind. They are not real. They are the product of your mind's evaluation of the situation. Except for the bears.

Negative thoughts and what to do with them

We cannot help it: our minds are always spinning and churning, always planning, evaluating, and agonizing, worrying about things that already happened and cannot be changed, or about things that will never happen. It is exhausting.

How do you get a grip on that constant roller-coaster of negative thoughts and emotions in your head?

Here are some simple exercises:

1. Move. Physical exercise encourages your body to produce endorphins; hormones that make us feel good. Moving also gets you out, away from the phone, Facebook, TV and the news, into nature. Go running, swimming, hiking, dancing, or any kind of exercise you enjoy. While you are doing it, your mind will stop the roller coaster of constant overanalyzing and worrying.

2. Enjoy your favorite music. Something cheerful, with a bit of a beat. Nothing serious or sad.

3. Learn about mindful meditation. There are clubs and YouTube videos to show you how to do it. It is worth the effort. Mindfulness teaches you to focus on the present moment and meditation teaches you to slow down your breathing and your mind, relax and get balanced. You will feel your tense muscles relax and you did not even know they were tense.

4. Learn to breathe, deep and slowly, filling your lungs with oxygen, which goes to all your parts, including your brain.

5. Laugh out loud until your stomach hurts and your eyes water. Watch a movie with friends, read a funny book. Laughing is another activity that boosts the production of good hormones.

Did you notice that these are the same exercises recommended as part of your self-care? You will hear more about them because those are simple exercises that ground you and force you to slow down your ever-spinning mind.

Building self-confidence – bringing out the best in you

Conquering your fears and learning how to control your emotions are just a few steps toward building your self-confidence.

We mentioned before that self-confidence is the way you perceive yourself, how you evaluate who you are, how you feel, and how you look and act. Being confident means feeling good about who you are, and being comfortable with yourself. Without self-confidence, you will not even think about changing the life you are not happy with, and surely not have the guts to actually change it.

Your confidence is your own estimate of who you are and what you are capable of. It is not always accurate and often not always the way other people see you.

Your confidence is fragile and it goes up and down in different situations. It depends on whether what happens confirms or denies your current belief about yourself. It is much more important what you think and believe about yourself than what other people think or believe about you, whether it is good or bad.

It is very important that you learn who you really are, your best qualities, and your likes and dislikes. It is difficult to be totally objective and honest with yourself, so you need help with that. Ask someone you trust, someone who knows you and loves you enough to help you with this self-evaluation. Once you have a better, realistic picture, you know what you have to work with.

According to psychologists, self-confidence has three elements:

Competence – your idea about your skills and effectiveness in any situation;

Resilience – how fast and how well you bounce back from any hardship that life throws at you; and

Optimism – whether you are hopeful that things will get better.

We are all different and we have different strengths and weaknesses. That is a good thing. Imagine if all people were the same. What a boring world that would be.

Do not forget that this is not about your abilities. It is about your belief in your abilities. Much more important.

Once you know with some certainty your level of self-confidence, there are exercises that can help you improve it. Do not need any improvement? You are a very rare, special person or you are not truthful with yourself.

1. Make a list of positive goals

This activity will help you understand that you are fully capable of achieving your goals.

Write a list of five goals you want to achieve. Make sure your goals are realistic and are within your power to achieve them. For example, "I will paint this bookshelf."

Make sure your goal is measurable ("I will finish painting the bookshelf by Friday."). The goal should also be relevant and have some meaning and importance for you (the bookshelf has to be done before your son comes back from the camping trip).

When you get into the spirit of this exercise, choose more challenging goals. Choose something that requires your brain, skills, and some serious effort. With practice, you will realize that you can do whatever task you have ahead of yourself if you put your will and your mind to it.

2. Overcome negative beliefs

Negative experiences make you doubt yourself and your abilities. To unveil and verify your negative beliefs about yourself, make a list of all your negative beliefs about yourself you can think of. Long list? Don't worry; most of them are only in your mind.

Show that list to someone who knows you, who you trust, and who loves you (your parents, friends or siblings). Ask them to write a comment next to each of your negative beliefs. Ask them to change these negative beliefs into realistic, constructive ones.

You will be amazed how many of your negative beliefs about yourself are exaggerated and overblown in importance.

You dropped a tray of drinks at the party? It does not make you a clumsy fool, just someone who tripped on the carpet or someone who should not wear high heels.

3. Appreciate yourself

Make a list of your good qualities. Cannot think of a single one? It happens when your self-confidence is low or you are doubting yourself. This list of questions will help:

What do I like about myself? (Combine diverse qualities like looks, character, achievements.)

Describe me in three words.

What are my skills and talents?

Show this list to your parents or friends and ask them to write down their list of your qualities.

Very different, right? It is more than likely that their list of your qualities is much longer than yours. It will tell you a lot about how those who know you and love you see you and just how low your self-image is.

4. Daily motivation

There are days when you do not feel like getting out of bed. But you have to. The trick is finding something that will motivate you to go through even the toughest day.

Find a pretty box and make it your "motivation box." Find some meaningful motivational quotes on the internet and write those you particularly like on a piece of paper. Fold each paper and put it in your "motivation box."

Each morning, before leaving the house, pick a random piece of paper and read aloud the motivation of the day. It will hopefully get you going through the day.

Remember, you are stronger and better than you are aware of. All you need to do is dig it out and bring it to the surface. Sometimes a piece of paper with a helpful, hopeful quote can make a big difference. Positive thinking is powerful.

Building resilience

Resilience is your inner ability to recover, to bounce back from the hardships you encounter. Life is always full of challenges. You cannot avoid them but you can prepare for them.

Some people prefer to avoid difficulties and hide from them. Staying home and doing nothing is one way. But then you hide from life as well. We spoke before about dealing with fear. This is the same: the best way to deal with challenges is to face them head-on.

You might get hurt, and you might suffer, but you will recover. How fast you recover from such encounters depends on how resilient you are. Often, being resilient is more important than being strong.

Here are some things that build resilience:

1.The power of love

If you were lucky, you were and are loved by your parents, family, friends, grandparents, neighbors, and your dog. That love is your first shield against the world and its hardships. Being loved means you are worth it and precious.

Not everyone is lucky to grow up in a loving environment. But we need love and you can encourage it and nurse it in those around you. Make a circle of friends that you can trust, that can support you while you support them, and who will love you for you, without judgment. Show that you care to other people, your care might encourage care and love in them.

2.Have high expectations

Those who love you have very high expectations of you. Not to have a lot of money, the best hair, the perfect apartment, powerful job. They expect you to have dignity, courage, compassion, empathy, and self-respect. You should have the same high expectations from yourself to be the best you can be.

3.Being resilient does not mean you will not get hurt

Resilience will not protect you from life's harsh realities. It will not protect you from being hurt at times. Being resilient means that you will recover faster and stronger from the experience. You will get hurt, but your resilience will help you to bounce back stronger every time you are challenged to your limits.

4.Practice self-care

Making a big change in your life will take everything you have, especially your health, mental and physical. If you do not take good care of yourself, you will not have the energy to make changes, your resilience will suffer and your immune system will be in danger, making you vulnerable to diseases. You will be more prone to depression and bouts of anxiety.

What self-care are we talking about? The one that you never had time for.

Self-care is "the practice of taking an active role in protecting one's well-being and happiness, in particular during periods of stress" (Oxford Dictionary).

You probably saw articles about self-care exercises and courses in the media. But it is actually very simple. Self-care means taking care of yourself and your physical and mental well-being, so that you are strong enough to deal with whatever hits you in life.

Self-care consists of habits you should develop and practice every day. Yes, every day. These habits are meant to support your health and well-being.

It is up to you to choose the activities that help you relax, unwind or de-stress. The difference is that you have to make them habits, something you do every day, just like brushing your teeth. You might try different things until you find a routine that you enjoy and which is not a chore.

Do not look for an excuse, such as not having enough time, being too busy, or considering these activities self-indulgence.

Taking care of your health and well-being is far from indulgence. It is necessary in order to keep you strong, healthy and resilient to make the changes you would like to make. Remember, creating new, good habits is part of those changes.

Start with just 15 minutes a day and increase it when you feel the need or particularly enjoy an activity (hiking in the woods might make you lose track of time).

What should be included in your daily routine?

Self-care means caring for all aspects of your health and well-being: physical, social, emotional, mental, and spiritual. Include something that will support all of your needs every day. Well-balanced exercises lower your feeling of anxiety, prevent depression, support your self-esteem, and make you more powerful, more in control and stronger.

Here are some elements that have to be part of your daily routine:

Do something physical

Ride a bike, walk the trails, dance, jump rope, swim, skate, and play basketball with friends; just get your heart beating and blood flowing.

Sleep at least 8 hours

Do not skimp on sleep. About eight hours of uninterrupted sleep is necessary for optimal health. If you do not sleep enough, you will be cranky, impatient, and lack focus and energy. Some people need less sleep. You know yourself best.

Learn yoga

There must be a yoga group or studio near you. Yoga is an ancient practice that offers both physical and spiritual benefits. Once you master basic exercises, you can do them at home, in your garden, or on the balcony. You will feel the benefit for the rest of your life. Yoga clubs are great places to meet new friends.

Get out

Get out into nature, look at the sky, smell the flowers, walk barefoot on the grass, and listen to the crickets. We are all part of nature, let it heal you.

Drink a lot of water

Stay hydrated, your body needs water to function properly. No coffee, no soda. Just clean water. Green tea is fine.

Eat well

Eat balanced, healthy meals. Provide your body with nutrients. Junk food is not food. Eat plenty of fresh fruits and vegetables.

Meditate

Mindful meditation is a thousand-year-old practice that will help you relax, reduce anxiety, lower stress and help you balance your body and mind.

Be grateful for what you have

As part of your daily routine, think of or write down three things you are currently grateful for. Think simple: your son called you from school, you managed to get that book you were looking for, or your boss complimented you on the last report. It is ok if you find more than three things.

Find something to believe in

Believing in something bigger than you makes you feel grounded. It can be God, nature, human goodness, or love.

Do random acts of kindness

Make someone's day better by smiling at them on the street, helping your neighbor in her garden, calling your parents, offer to help in the soup kitchen, etc. Open yourself up to the world. If you make your world bigger, your troubles will look smaller.

Meet people

Even if you are an introvert, you need people. We are tribal creatures. We need to surround ourselves with other people to feel human. You have the right to avoid toxic people, even if they are your family. Choose people who make you smile, laugh, or feel safe.

Give yourself a gift

Sometimes, you need to do something for yourself that is not a reward and not something you need. Indulge yourself in a visit to the hairdresser, buy a new book, go to a concert, or have a fancy dinner.

Do something artistic

Unleash your inner artist, dig those crayons or paints out, mold some clay, knit a scarf, or play with Photoshop.

Walk your dog

Some activities combine more than one benefit. Walking a dog is one of them. You get the exercise, the unconditional love and gratitude of your dog, and you spend some time in nature. There is no end to the benefits of having a dog.

You now get the idea of activities that should comprise your self-care. Nothing different from what you are doing anyway. But when you do them consciously, aware of their importance, every day, you will soon see the benefits. And they will last you a lifetime.

Boosting willpower

You might have the best intentions, but if you do not have the willpower, nothing will happen. The lack of willpower can sabotage our best plans and leave our most important goals in the dust.

Willpower is defined as a control over doing something or not doing it. It is also defined as power to resist impulses.

It is easy to say, "Oh, my willpower is lousy, I can never resist a new pair of shoes," or "I do not have willpower to wake up early enough to go for a run." Basically, it is a copout. It can prevent you from making better habits and getting rid of bad ones. It will sabotage your effort to make meaningful differences in your life. So, can you improve your willpower? Of course, but you have to want to.

Instant gratification vs. long term goal

We learn as kids to do the homework first in order to get cookies later. But as we get older, we become greedy and want instant gratification all the time. It is one reason why it is so difficult to make drastic changes in your life.

A lot of the comfort you are used to will be at risk; your bad habit that kept you living the life that is not making you happy will have to be trashed; your need to please everyone by becoming everyone's darling, but not your own, will have to be replaced with better habits. But for that, you have to have willpower.

Poor willpower is what makes us take one more glass of wine, or another steak, or watch another episode on

Netflix. Poor willpower also makes us have hard time saying 'no' to a bully friend or dominating husband, or spoiled children.

Willpower is the effort to resist all short-term temptations in order to meet long-term goals. You can look at it as a struggle between logic, what makes sense, and emotions. You know that spending the next hour studying will ensure you a better grade tomorrow, but you really want to watch one more episode of your favorite show.

If you are struggling with resisting temptations and wish to have more willpower to do the right things, here are some exercises to help you:

Go slowly, don't take too much all at once. Divide each goal into small, manageable tasks. If you want to lose weight, start by cutting down on snacks and sugary sodas. You do not have to start the new exercise regime by spending an hour in the gym every day. You will get discouraged in no time. Start by short walks and increase the time by ten minutes every day.

Always plan ahead. When you make decisions about what to do in advance, you help your willpower to resist deviating from the plan and giving in to temptations. If eating healthy is your goal, make a weekly menu and get all necessary ingredients in advance. Get a treat as well, so you do not have irresistible cravings. If you spend money on high quality ingredients, you will be less tempted to stop by a fast food place. If drinking too much is your issue, do not hang out with your gang in a bar after work. Go with a friend who will support your decision to have only one glass of wine or only one cocktail.

Stay away from temptation. If you have hard time resisting fatty foods, do not keep them in your fridge. If you are going to eat in a restaurant, go to a vegetarian place, or choose fish. If you are trying to stay away from alcohol, do not keep any of it at home, and avoid parties where you know there will be a lot of drinking.

When you are tired and stressed, your willpower is at an all-time low. Strengthen it with mindfulness meditations and enough sleep.

Mark important milestones with a reward. Every time you reach a milestone on your way to reaching your goal, celebrate. If you lost 40 pounds, buy a lovely new dress. If you passed an exam in your night school, buy that book you were coveting. If you managed to finish a half-marathon, treat yourself with a visit to the hairdresser.

Find your tribe. Hang out with like-minded people. Join a hiking group, find a neighbor who wants to go running with you in the morning, ask your kids to join your new vegetarian diet. Whatever your goal is, there are people who have a similar goal or are just willing to support you. They are your tribe.

Chapter 5

Defining Success

Albert Schweitzer wrote "Success is not the key to happiness. Happiness is the key to success..." Defining success is as difficult as defining happiness and you will find as many definitions as there are people you ask. Is success necessary for happiness? What really is success? Most articles you can find equate success with a successful career and business. But when you look at the definition of success, you will find something very different:

English Language dictionary defines success as " the accomplishment of an aim or purpose." Now, this is more like it. Now the words of Albert Schweitzer make sense. Because what you consider success might be totally irrelevant to someone else. And even more importantly, what you consider success today might be very different from what you meant by success when you were young.

Success in midlife

Men think that women define success in terms of a good relationship and balanced life, while men require financial and career accomplishments to consider themselves successful. How wrong they are. They must be thinking about some women from the romantic era. We want it all.

Remember when you were in your 20s, you wanted to get a highly-paid job that would give you the power to fulfill your vision? You wanted a career that would make tabloids write about you. You wanted a big wedding to the love of your life. And to find that love of your life, of course. You wanted a couple of kids but were not sure if you should wait until your career has peaked. You wanted a big house, a fancy car, and a glamorous wardrobe.

Then life came and you grew up. It is not that all those things were not achievable for you. Many probably were. But as you grew older, many of them became less important.

What happened? You learned that the old saying "Be careful what you wish for" is true. You learned that financial success came with sacrifices you made then but would not make now. You learned that there are many things that were not even on your list of 'desirable in order to be successful,' but are all of sudden the reason you see your life as unsuccessful.

You met your expectations and fulfilled all your previous criteria for success, but your expectations changed.

When you reach your infamous midlife crisis, your definition of success needs revising. Whether you achieved what you wanted in your 20s or not, you are now starting from the new definition of success, from the new goals that you need to achieve in order to consider yourself successful.

Your new definition of success in business

If you were lucky to get the career in the field you wanted early in life, your new definition is to get the best at it as you can be, to make your career meaningful, and to serve as more than just financial success. You want to continue learning and to open new paths and discuss new ideas. You want to mentor other women in choosing their career path.

You might discover that what you considered a desirable career in your 20s, becoming a lawyer or accountant, did not fulfill your need. It maybe gave you financial success but it forced you to forget your dreams.

And now, in your 40s and 50s, you are afraid that if you do not do something about those dreams, you never will. You know that you would be a much better painter than an accountant. You are sure that your dream to be a fashion designer would lead to some spectacular clothes even if it never puts you on the covers of fashion magazines.

If you never had a career and had to accept any job that paid the bills early on, your dreams are much bigger. You want that career other women had years to develop. You want to be a lawyer because you always dreamed about justice and fighting for the marginalized. You want to work to fulfill your passion and not just for the salary.

So what do you do? You see what you have to work with and make a plan. You might have to go back to school. Or look for a more challenging position in your company. If you are the boss, you might want to hire some talented people with a vision to help you change the path of your company.

Or you might have to quit and find your dream job. If you can afford it. That is the time when you really have to evaluate what you have to work with: are you trained and skilled for your dream job? Do you have enough money to survive until you get your dream job? Can you count on help and support from your spouse or partner? You do not want your family to suffer from your decision to go after your dream.

Your new definition of success in a romantic relationship

If you got married in your 20s and 30s, you might have lucked out and ended up in a healthy, solid relationship that survived all hardship and got only stronger. Such a partner will be your solid rock when going through the turmoil of a midlife crisis.

But not all of us are that lucky. If you found out that the man you married is not making you happy, and is in fact making you miserable, now is the time to decide what to do. If you do not, you will end up spending the rest of your life in an unsatisfactory relationship. Unless he leaves you in your 50s with no alimony, no career, lonely and miserable.

You have options. You can adapt. You can learn to be more flexible and accept some of your partner's more irritating habits. You can go for marriage counseling. You can have a good, honest talk and create some boundaries.

Or you can get a divorce. In that case, make sure you get a good lawyer.

If you are in the position to look for a new partner in your 40s and 50s, you will be looking for a very different person than you did in your 20s. Looks will not be too important. You will be looking for compatibility in all aspects, from your values to interests and temperament.

You will be looking for someone financially stable because you are not going to put another man through school. You will have to learn how to navigate treacherous dating sites, or trust old-fashioned "friend of the friend" help. Or join a club you are interested in. You are hoping to meet someone you will spend the rest of your life with, so don't rush.

Your new definition of success in life

This one is not easy and trying to answer it will help you re-evaluate your goals for a better life. It deserves some deep thinking and one way to do it is to write it down.

Try to write down everything that comes to your mind without bothering with grammar or composition. Free-flow writing takes into account things that come from your intuition, emotions, past experiences, and your gut.

Make it simple and natural. Give yourself five minutes to describe what you mean by success. Start each line with "Success is..." Then complete the sentence with whatever spontaneously comes to your mind. Don't think too hard. Let it flow.

Now, have a look at your list and think about your criteria for a successful life. Are some of them superficial, such as "...to have a lot of money," or "I want a big house." Are you sure that is really what would make you successful, and happy? If you did not have those things, could you still be happy?

What are your deal-breakers? What are the conditions that are absolutely necessary for being successful in life? Those are things you have to focus on when making plans for the changes in your life.

Small can be big

You do not have to go for monumental changes to achieve success. It just has to be a success in achieving any goal you set for yourself. If your goal is to learn Chinese so you can teach English as a second language, achieving that will give you an enormous sense of accomplishment and lead you toward a successful, exciting new career.

The more you push yourself to achieve your goal, the bigger sense of success you will feel. Trying new things, facing your fears and overcoming old roadblocks are sure signs of success.

Chasing old goals

Like the rest of us, you must have painful memories of the goals you had when you were younger but were not successful in achieving. Now, in your 40s and 50s, you are in a very different place. Are those goals still important to you? If they are, consider going after them now. You are older, wiser, more confident and have more experience.

You know that you are still the same woman as before, but you might be more ready for achieving that success that eluded you when you were younger now.

Don't think for a moment that it is too late to start something new and big. Consider all those wonderful women who did not achieve success until later years.

It is never too late

Achieving success in your midlife is not as rare as you would think. National Bureau of Economic Research found that twice as many 50-year-old entrepreneurs started successful high-growth firms than those in their 30s.

Laura Ingalls Wilder published her first book "Little House Big Wood" when she was 65.

Vera Wang started thinking about her own business designing wedding gowns when she was 40.

Toni Morrison published her first book when she was 40. Until then, she was a hard-working single mom.

Ann Dowd achieved success in her middle 50s. She has some advice for all women looking at new beginnings: "Stay humble. Stay grateful. Believe in yourself. Have unshakeable faith in yourself."

Most wise successful women say that what we see as a sudden brilliant success has behind it years and even decades of preparation. Maybe your preparations are over and you are ready to jump feet-first into that big new adventure. What if you do not succeed? You will not know if you do not try.

Another wise thing successful women say is to insist on staying who you are, but real, authentic you, sticking to your passions and you will succeed in whatever you put your mind to. You do not need anyone's permission.

When you were young, it was so important to please everyone, to have external recognition to feel worthy. Now you do not care so much about what anyone thinks. Only what you feel is right.

Do not wait for just the right time to do it perfectly. That time might never come. Choose progress, slow steady progress, making things better over perfection.

Choose your tribe

There is no need to do it alone. Find other women who are on the same path toward success as you are. In fact, they will probably find you. Make them into your tribe. You have all been underestimated and marginalized, failed so many times that you do not feel pain anymore. You have each other, to encourage, to pull out of bouts of negative thoughts and doubts.

You must have seen advice that you should stop being a victim and become a predator. Is this really what you have to become? That mentality is what is making our world so mean and people so vicious to each other.

On the contrary. In your midlife, you know the power of encouragement, of empathy and understanding. You are not competing with each other. There is enough space in the world for many successful, happy, fulfilled women. Lift each other up, do not push each other down.

Small changes are changes too

Reading about successful older women makes you think that success is about running big corporations, starting your own business, or becoming a household name. Most of us do not crave this kind of success.

What we want is to make what we have better.

Not everyone has big dreams. Many of us do not need drastic changes to feel happier. Most of us cannot move to Costa Rica and open an eco-hotel. We have kids and old parents to take care of. But we do want our job to mean something. We want our partner to treat us with love and respect. We want more time to spend with friends. We want an opportunity to express our artistic side.

Nobody has a prescription for a more successful life. You are the only one who can decide what it is that will make you happier. And what is within your reach. It would be counterproductive to start feeling inadequate because you are not ready to turn your life upside down, but just want to make it better. You go after your goals, not anyone else's.

Good habits of successful people

To be successful in whatever goal you pursue requires strong drive, a passion for your goal, and some good habits. We have already discussed the need to establish some good habits in your pursuit of happiness and to get rid of some bad ones that were holding you back. Here are some habits highly successful people consider crucial:

Getting up early

Most successful people consider it necessary to get up about three hours before their work day starts. They use that time to plan the day ahead, to exercise, do a few personal chores and just breathe and focus. These three hours give them time to start the day without a mad rush and stress before they even begin. Wake up with the sun, start slowly, gather your strength and start with a purpose.

Reading a lot is necessary

To succeed in any endeavor, you need to keep up with what is happening, stay updated with the latest developments in your field and work on improving your skills.

While reading for pleasure is not a crucial part of business success, it is necessary for your well-being. Give yourself at least 15 minutes a day to immerse yourself in a good novel, in some self-improving lecture, or a biography of a person you admire.

Focus

Things happen fast during the day. You often act on auto-pilot in order to accomplish everything you have to, from work tasks to family obligations to keeping in touch with family and friends. You need to stop at some point and process all that.

You need at least 15 minutes to spend alone, to focus on everything that is going on and process it. Depending on your lifestyle, you can choose to do it early morning before your day starts, or in the evening, when all your chores are done and you are ready to go to sleep.

Try to tackle all aspects of your life: a project you are working on, relationships with colleagues, family issues, kids' problems, your health and feelings. While you are focusing, try to slow your breathing and relax your muscles. If you have some time, end your focus time with a bit of meditation. Empty your mind and focus only on breathing.

Having time to process what is happening greatly reduces your stress because it helps you get prepared for what is coming.

Exercise is crucial

It is interesting how many rich and successful people give exercise a priority. They find that regular exercise helps them clear their mind and improves their motivation.

Choose an exercise you enjoy. Ideally, do something that will take you out into nature: jogging, walking, or biking. Many successful people find that exercise not only take their valuable time from work but, in fact, it also improves their productivity.

Again, some people prefer to exercise in the morning, just after waking up. Others like to get out after work, distress and clear their mind while moving their muscles. If you have a dog, you have to do both, for the dog's benefit, but for your own as well.

Spend time with someone who inspires you

If you want to stay motivated, socialize with other motivated people. Hanging out with people that encourage your bad habits does not help. If you know people who are positive, focused and motivated, spend as much time with them as you can.

They do not have to be in your business circle. People who volunteer and devote part of their time to helping others are highly motivated and are great to spend time with. Join a soup kitchen, community garden, or any volunteer group in your neighborhood. It will do you good to spend some time helping others, but people you will meet will become part of your support team, even if they are gardeners, chefs, or church pastors.

Get enough sleep

Not everyone needs the same amount of sleep to function optimally, but there is a necessary minimum. You know yourself. Most people need about eight hours of uninterrupted sleep.

During sleep, you are resting your body and mind, but your mind is using that time to store long-term memories.

If you are wondering when you can find those eight hours when you already have to get up three hours before work to exercise and plan your day, think about the time you spend doing frivolous and time-wasting things such as checking your Facebook or other social media accounts. Or watching some mindless show on TV. It is fine to check your social media accounts, but you know very well how easy it is to go on a tangent and spend hours browsing stupid comments.

If you know people you admire and who are successful in whatever they are pursuing, whether it is mastering piano playing, learning Chinese or starting a new business, talk to them. Ask them about habits they consider important for their success.

Chapter 6

Evaluating expectations

Unhappy with your lot? Social scientists say that it is normal in your 40s and 50s. Is this supposed to make you feel better? No, but it might make you feel less guilty and miserable. You are going through a stage in life in which you question what you have done with your life so far and you find it lacking. You feel like you have failed. Have you really? Let's talk about one big obstacle to your happiness at this age: Expectations.

How unrealistic expectations sabotage your happiness

Like all good girls, you have followed your parents' and society's map for a happy life: you went to school, got a diploma, got a job, became financially independent, got married, got a couple of kids, and bought a house. Now you are saying that is not enough? You knew that many of your school friends were not as lucky and took different, less successful paths. But that was no consolation to you.

The problem is that this map is mostly not working. It is made for some perfect people who do not exist. You might have dropped out of school when you got pregnant. You married a high school sweetheart but he fell in love with his secretary and left you and the kids. The job you got is mind-bogglingly boring but it pays the bills. Taking kids through school is expensive so you are constantly struggling with money.

So your expectations that if you only follow the plan you will have a happy life, failed. But that does not mean that you failed.

You have to accept that not everything is in your power. Circumstances, other people, economic inequality, and some bad decisions brought you to this point in life. And you are not happy. And you really want to be happy.

So, what to do? The first thing to do is ask yourself: what is it that I really want? What would make me happier? Powerful career? To marry George Clooney? To have a big house with a swimming pool?

Let's get real. If those were your expectations when you were 20, no wonder you are not happy for not achieving them. Almost nobody could. Except for that gorgeous lawyer who snagged George.

Does this mean that you cannot be happy? Not at all. You just have to rein in your expectations a bit and evaluate what happiness really means.

Happiness in the 40s

Until now, you have been living your life building it, working on it, in the hope that all that work will pay off and one day you will be happy. And now you realize that you have wasted so much time because it did not work. You are unhappy. Instead of enjoying every day of your life, you were living for that distant future when elusive happiness will arrive.

In the meantime, you have lost the opportunity to be happy with what you already had. Scientists say that after midlife crisis things get better. We stop living for the future and start living for the present. But that is no consolation to you right now.

The recipe for happiness

The best way to find out whether it is possible to be happy at this stage of your life is to ask people who consider themselves happy what their secret is. What is it that they do that makes them happy? And you will find out that you were looking for all the wrong things.

Take care of meaningful relationships

Your career, the kids, and endless chores probably forced you to neglect your friends and family. Chasing financial success did not leave much time for hanging out with people who you care for and who make you happy every time you meet them.

But when a crisis strikes, those are the people you turn to. They are the shoulders you cry on, people who lend you money when you are broke and babysit your kids when you need help. They are your support system, but they are also a constant, unwavering source of happiness. Just think about what life would look like if they were not in it.

So nurture those relationships. Find time for your friends, regardless of how tired you are after work. Remember their birthdays, have lunches with them and enjoy laughing out loud and being surrounded by happiness.

The older you get, the more you appreciate that relationships in your life matter much more than your career or financial success.

The most important relationship

If you are lucky and you have been married or in a long-term relationship for a while now, how is that working? Do you feel taken for granted? But aren't you doing the same to him? He grew a beer belly and some weird mustache? But what about your wrinkles and sagging boobs?

If he is still attentive, a good father, brings home a salary to take care of the family, and never forgets your birthday, there is still love there. It is time to rekindle that passion that once existed. Love is a powerful force and has the ability to make you utterly miserable but also deliriously happy.

Keep in mind that your husband or partner is probably also going through a midlife crisis. Talk about it and help each other. Try to laugh about it, it has its funny side. Revive that love. Now that the kids are gone, you have the whole house to yourself. You have the opportunity to play. And play is the best way to rekindle that monotonous, routine sex. Don't be shy to bring in sex toys, videos, and lubricants, and there is a good reason why Viagra is the most popular pill in the world.

If you are thinking of making some big changes in your life, making them with your partner would be so much easier. Compromise if your dreams are different and if your risk-adversity is not the same.

Find time for your hobbies

Your career might be unsatisfactory and you might be doing a job that you do only because you need that salary at the end of the month. But, there are things you really enjoy doing. Spend time on your hobbies. You were not able to make a career of your painting, but it does not mean that you cannot pour your creativity onto a canvas from time to time. That is also part of who you are, and it will give you happiness.

Give up unrealistic expectations.

By now you know your strengths and weaknesses. You are becoming more realistic about what you can achieve and what you really cannot, regardless of your dreams. Once you accept this, you will feel less stressed and stop expecting the impossible from yourself. So what if you did not fulfill your dreams from your 20s. You knew so little about yourself at that age and what you are capable of, and what you are not.

And it is not always about you. Often, it is about circumstances. You envy your friend who quit her job and went to volunteer in Cambodia. But her kids were grown up and had their own jobs, she divorced her husband, and she was free. You are not. Your kids are still dependent on you, you love your husband with all his limitations and you are not ready or willing to leave the family and friends that make your world.

So you cannot save the world? There is so much you can do about saving the world without going to Cambodia. In your own town, in your own neighborhood. You do not have to give up your aspirations, you just have to make them more realistic.

Share your misery with friends

Understanding what is happening and why you are feeling so restless in your 40s and 50s helps you to deal with it. It also helps to realize that you are not alone in it and that many of your friends are going through the same turmoil. You are not the failure and your sense of being disappointed with yourself is a normal effect of this transitional period of your life.

Talk to your friends about it. Exchange experiences. Laugh about the misery that is making you so constantly anxious and often depressed. Get some good wine and trash your other friends who are doing plastic surgery to feel younger and starting to look like Stepford Wives. Exchange tips on dealing with the crisis and help each other where you can. Sometimes taking a friend who is feeling depressed to a spa can make a difference in her life, and will surely make you feel good too.

Enjoy every moment

When you were younger, the future looked far away and you felt that you had all the time in the world to achieve what you wanted. Now that half of your life is gone, you realize that you do not have any time to waste to be happy.

The future is here, so make the best of it. Make every moment an opportunity to be happy. That is why people over 60 are so much happier, as long as their health is still good. They know that they have little time left, so they might as well enjoy every day.

You do not have to abandon your goals, but accept that the goals have changed. To achieve happiness, you have to reevaluate what makes you happy. You are now looking for more meaning in what you do and less financial success. You create goals that are easier to achieve but are not less fulfilling.

So what if you did not follow the traditional path and did not get married and did not get kids? So what if you did not create an important career but followed your heart running a garden center, which did not fill your wallet but did fill your heart. There are so many different paths to happiness.

Appreciate what you have

Positive people are always happier, so kill that inner critic and look at what you have instead of what you do not have. No big house? But you have a lovely small house you've already paid off. No fancy car? Your bike takes you places and offers great exercise. No big office and powerful position? Being a teacher has much more opportunity for making a big change in the world; you are creating future world leaders.

One good way to appreciate what you have is to volunteer. Go help those less fortunate and it will make you humble and much more appreciative of what you have. Go volunteer in the local hospital and see what it means to be sick and have your whole life taken away from you.

Rediscover nature

The Covid pandemic did a serious number on us, but it taught us many important lessons. It completely changed our idea of what is important. It also taught us that we have a hard time living without a connection with nature. Not being able to go out became a very big issue.

We keep forgetting that we are animals. Sophisticated, complicated animals, but nevertheless, a part of nature. We need that connection and our urban life mostly deprived us of it.

You must have read about what nature means for lowering stress and helping with depression. Nature means being surrounded by plants and animals and using all our senses to enjoy the world around us. Does nature make you feel small and insignificant? It should not. It should make you feel like a part of something bigger and majestic.

So get out, breathe deeply, touch the trees, listen to the birds. But also help nurture that nature, our lives depend on it. Plant a tree, protect those endangered turtles, take care of your garden. Nature will make you smile without any reason and will make you happy for just being.

Don't go there

It is common in this age to keep returning to the dark places: past mistakes, hurt we caused to someone, self-doubt, poor judgments, rage, dreams of revenge, and deep hate. Do not go there. It is counterproductive, useless, exhausting, and toxic. Every time you feel your mind is taking you in that direction, tell yourself not to go there, you are done with it.

Learn to do nothing

Doing nothing in your busy life feels like an indulgence. And who has time for it, anyway. But it is necessary and it might take you some time to learn how to do it. The official name for this activity is meditation, but you can also call it total relaxation, deep breathing, or whatever. It consists of emptying your mind as much as you can. Just try not to think; let your senses bring in feelings. Try to hear the sound of the wind, crickets chirping, birds singing, the ocean crashing, and your own heart beating. Every time you feel your thoughts intruding, snap out of it and go back to what the senses are bringing you. Give your mind a break.

De-clutter your life

You know how clutter in your home drives you crazy and does not allow you to relax? Your mind can also get cluttered. It is always churning, processing, and storing. It is full of all kinds of stuff and the new stuff keeps coming in. And all that stuff competes for our attention. The result? Total mind clutter. No wonder we feel like we cannot focus, we cannot function well, and we are always stressed and unhappy.

Unfortunately, we cannot send our mind clutter to the Salvation Army together with old clothes and furniture. What we can do is sift through all that clutter and get rid of excess, pretty much the way you do with other stuff.

Start small. Acknowledge that you have a problem. Once you are aware of it, you can deal with it.

With so many things competing for your attention, you need to prioritize, choose the things that matter most and focus on them. Abandon others or push them to the bottom of the line. Life is short.

You need to acknowledge that sometimes you need help. When you are overwhelmed with too many competing responsibilities and obligations, you need to find someone who knows how to listen, and who will let you talk about everything until things are clearer. If you are lucky to have a partner you can do it with, you are a lucky woman. A very good friend is fine too, but they are not easy to find either.

Get rid of toxic people

This is not easy but it can make a difference between misery and happiness. There are people that are making you unhappy but are a part of our life: relatives, colleagues, and so-called friends. Every time you are in their company, they drain your energy and make you feel bad about yourself. They are always there to point out that your hair is a mess, or that you really messed up with that report.

However hard it is, you need to get them out of your life. If it means not going to family gatherings, so be it. Moving to another department of your company or even changing company is sometimes necessary. The more important their role is, the more important it is to separate them from your life. If it is a boss, it might mean looking for another job. If it is a spouse, it might mean a divorce.

It is not easy but what a relief when it is done! You owe it to yourself to get rid of as much negativity in your life as possible. Why should you let anyone prevent you from being happy? It is difficult enough as it is.

Chapter 7

Empowerment is the best fuel

Did you notice a subtle thread that weaves through all the chapters? It is about your perception of yourself. We discussed the issue of midlife crisis and how to respond to it. We discussed happiness, what it means and how to achieve it.

We also talked about how to be successful in reaching all your goals; the empowerment and the tools you need in order to reach your goals on your way to a more meaningful and happier life.

In the previous chapter, we addressed the big obstacle to your happiness created by your unrealistic expectations.

But what if you are not willing to be limited by any of it? If your drive to make a change to your life after reaching midlife is strong and powerful? If what to others looks like unrealistic expectations is not unrealistic to you?

If you are not willing to give up your big dreams, and you are sure that you are confident, empowered, and resilient to go through all the obstacles to reaching your goals, then nothing can stand in your way.

Except for a few small things, among them the fact that life will sap you occasionally of your now so-strong motivation. Let's deal with that right away.

Motivation

Motivation is a force, an internal process that makes you do things and move toward your goal. Women have a perpetual motivation in their need to take care of the kids and family. Powerful motivation will make you develop some good habits that will help you in all aspects of your life.

When you are not motivated, any task looks difficult and any obstacle insurmountable. You are not looking forward to it and approach any goal with dread and anxiety. You feel like you are not capable of dealing with it.

What causes poor motivation?

There is a hidden underlying origin to our lack of motivation. While motivation varies from one moment to another and from one situation to another, some events in our lives or some negative beliefs we carry within us can cause us to lose motivation. Like:

- Perceived or real failures in the past;
- Unsupportive, unloving parents;
- Anxiety or depression;
- Negative beliefs about our own abilities;
- A lack of sleep;
- Procrastination habit;
- Non-existent self-accountability;
- Unrealistic and unachievable expectations;

- A stressful, unhealthy environment;
- Poor self-esteem.

What are the most powerful motivational forces for women?

Changing the world

We are all different but we all have some characteristics written in our genetic code: we are designed to nurture and care. We run not only our families but our society and our countries, often behind the scenes. We are changing the world one child at a time, one job, and one task at a time. This need to bring a meaningful change in the world by making small, everyday changes is a powerful force.

Trying new things

Visiting new places, trying a new game, new sport, or new challenge is exhilarating and highly motivating. Women thrive when they have the opportunity to spread their wings and challenge themselves. Even failure when trying new things is not an obstacle, just a challenge.

Achieving big goals

Achieving something big, overcoming a milestone or a big challenge is very empowering and highly motivating. The higher the goals women set for themselves, the bigger high they achieve when they make it. And the more successful they are, the more motivated they are to reach new heights.

Being respected

Being respected for what they do and what they stand for is a huge need and a strong motivator. The more we care for people, the more we crave their respect. Whatever women achieve, they need it to be recognized and respected by those they love, care for and respect in return. That is why it is so important to be surrounded by people whose opinions we value and whose respect matters to us. They motivate us to reach higher and higher.

Independence

Historically, women have been dependent on their families and spouses for everything they needed. That is the reason why being independent is so important for self-esteem and motivation. Being able to achieve something on their own, with their own abilities and strength is enormously motivating to women.

Taking care of themselves

Being able to take care of their body and mind is another big motivator for women. Having enough time to devote to their own needs means replenishing resources of energy and maintaining a strong and healthy body to deal with all obstacles. Self-care makes women feel good about themselves and motivated to deal with anything life throws at them.

Being challenged

Women thrive when faced with challenges and overcome them. That builds self-confidence to accept even bigger challenges and grow in power and ability to deal with obstacles. Challenges make us believe in ourselves and become motivated to deal with anything. Failing when faced with challenges is not a reason for self-doubt but a way to re-evaluate and learn from experience.

Breaking barriers

Throughout history and throughout their lives, women are always forced to face barriers and obstacles. Being able to break barriers by showing just how much they are capable of and how far from the stereotypes of soft and weaker sex they are.

Every time they break one barrier, women feel justified and encouraged to break more of them. Doing the jobs that were historically meant as men's jobs is one barrier women are breaking every day. From being pilots, astronauts, welders, and divers to company presidents and inventors, women have proven that there is no barrier they cannot overcome.

For women, breaking barriers is motivated not only by their own wish to succeed but also to pave the path for their daughters and granddaughters.

How to get motivated

The more we know ourselves, the better we are able to recognize signs that, for some reason, our motivation is low. We can look at what is causing it and address the problem. There are also some general tips for dealing with those situations when you feel that your motivation needs a boost.

Listen to your favorite mood-boosting song

Music can make us cry and laugh. It can lift our spirits or drown us in despair. We can use that power of music over our emotions to pick up pieces of music that are empowering and encouraging when we are in throes of self-doubt and feeling unmotivated to do anything.

You know your taste in music. Create a collection of songs that motivate you and keep them handy in times of need. Then give yourself a break to just listen and breathe.

A mood-lifting vision board

Just like with music, we can use photos, pictures, pieces of art, plants, and quotes that motivate us and lift our spirits to get out of the occasional funk. Make a vision board you can look at and quickly pick up bits of encouragement or even just a smile. A funny caricature, a photo of your puppy, or your last vacation can make you move from a negative to a positive frame of mind. Add to that any visible proof of your success like diplomas or a photo of you finishing a marathon.

It is easy to lose motivation when you are tired and feel like nothing is working. You need to remind yourself that it is just a temporary setback and not the reason for you to lose your motivation and belief in your abilities.

Get rid of those fears and insecurities

We all have deeply ingrained insecurities, fears and doubts that occasionally lift their ugly heads and cause us to lose motivation. You need to remind yourself that self-doubt is all in your head. It is not real proof of your lack of abilities. You have a lifetime of achievements to prove it.

Because those underlying insecurities can be powerful obstacles to achieving our goals, we need to acknowledge them in order to deal with them. Do you deep down think that you are just a housewife and not capable of running your own small online business? Do you secretly believe that you are a fraud and that at any moment everyone will discover just how little you know?

We all have those, but they are in our heads. Look at them honestly and laugh in their face. They are not real. They were created in the time of your self-doubts and it is time to get rid of them. You have earned it.

Look for a mentor

We all need someone we respect and admire who can take us out of our gloom and doom moments. When you are going through times when nothing seems to be working and whatever you touch seems to be failing, you need someone who will force you to look at things more objectively.

Often, it is enough that the mentor or advisor is just there to listen to you vent. Because most of the time you have a solution in your head but need to vocalize it or explain it to someone else to see it from another perspective.

Sometimes you need professional help. You might need help with marketing, or an engineer or a designer. You do not have to know everything but you need to know when to look for help.

Keep learning

Self-confidence is greatly based on our belief in our competence. Whatever task we have ahead of us, it is necessary to have enough knowledge to do it. With such fast development of science and technology, we need to constantly learn and research in order to have the latest information we need to complete the task. Constant education is the key to lasting self-confidence and motivation to strive for ever-bigger challenges.

Even when it comes to everyday life, knowing what is going on around us is crucial to feeling an active part of our community. The kids come from school with complex questions and we need to be able to answer them if we want to keep being their heroes.

Be aware of progress and success

Being aware of your achievements and progress will assure you of your abilities and worth. Keep a constant review of what you are doing and what you are achieving in all fields of your life. Celebrate successes and milestones, even the small ones. They are all steps towards your biggest goals. And nothing boosts motivation more than success.

Tell yourself that you are great

Women are especially prone to self-doubts and negative thoughts and self-talk. It is worse than having someone constantly bugging us and telling us that we suck. Make sure to eliminate negative words from your vocabulary and tell yourself that you are great. It is more important than when someone else tells you that.

And if you have people around you who never have a nice word to say, stay away from them. It is more about them than about you.

Announce your goals

Publicly announcing your goals is a great motivator and will force you to avoid procrastination. You will also have outside monitors and quality control. As long as those you are surrounded with are your kind of people, those who respect you and whose opinions matter to you.

Start with small tasks

When working on a large project, whether at work or building a house or making a dress, you might lose your motivation from stress, lack of time or just because it looks too overwhelming. Dividing a large task into smaller ones and completing each small task separately will give you a sense of going forward and accomplishing your task. And that brings motivation for the other parts of the project until it is all completed.

When you are going through periods of self-doubt and your motivation is low, give yourself some small, easily achievable tasks to feel better about yourself. It might be as small as planting some flowers into a pretty pot for your porch or baking a special cake.

Find some motivational speech that resonates with you

Motivational speakers are professionals who know just what to say to boost your self-confidence and improve your motivation. Listen to a few of them until you find one that resonates with you. Some of them are too corny but some are great.

The cup should always be half full

It might be in your nature to look at the glass as always half empty, but that is something you have to fight. A positive outlook improves your chance of having a positive outcome. Often, it is just a matter of perspective. You can see rain as bad weather or you can see it as great for the garden. You cannot control outside events but you can control how you evaluate them.

Look on the bright side

Try to find a funny side to any situation. Do not take yourself so seriously. Finding a bright side to a situation, regardless of how serious, helps deal with difficulties when they come. Everything can be overcome with a bit of courageous spirit and a dose of humor. Even if you make a mistake and things do not work well, make fun of the situation and yourself and the problem will not look so bad.

Keep the clutter under control

Clutter in your environment, at work and at home, adds to the daily stress. You have a hard time finding things, the chaos makes you out of control and the mess around you makes you feel like it is a reflection of the mess in your head. Get organized, declutter your space and keep it clean.

Don't share your plans with everyone

Successful people are in a habit of not revealing their plans to everyone out of fear that their ideas will be stolen. But even if you do not have a big, valuable idea, if you talk about your plans to everyone around you, someone might take your idea and present it as her or his own.

Or they might tell you and everyone else that it is bad, that it has no chance of succeeding or that you are out of your depth. All that can destroy your self-confidence and has nothing to do with reality. Be careful who you trust.

Surround yourself with happy and successful people

Successful and happy people have a contagious confidence that will boost your own. They create a positive environment around them and remind you that success and happiness are within your reach. In addition, successful people are a source of advice and a good influence.

Motivation is not something you can take for granted. It has to be renewed and boosted because it goes up and down with life. But the more self-confident you are, the longer lasting it is.

The power of positive thinking

Positive thinking is so powerful that there is an entire branch of psychology devoted to researching it. Earlier in this chapter, we tackled positive thinking as a way to deal with difficult situations and to be better motivated. But, positive thinking plays a much bigger role in our quest for happiness, so we need to examine it in more detail.

It seems that we are by nature prone to positive or negative thinking. Positive-thinking people approach challenges with a positive attitude or outlook.[2] They are not ignoring life's difficulties and challenges by seeing everything through 'rose-tinted glasses' as the expression goes. They just choose to always look at the obstacles as challenges and try to make the most of any bad situation. They always see the best in people and themselves.

Psychologists call it 'explanatory style':

People with an optimistic explanatory style freely take credit for good things when they happen and tend to blame some outside forces when things go bad. For them, negative happenings are temporary and are not typical.

People with a pessimistic explanatory style tend to blame themselves when bad things happen and do not give themselves enough credit for their successes. For them, when things go wrong, they are expected and constant. They blame themselves even for things that are totally out of their control.

How positive thinking affects health

The research shows that there are some concrete health benefits that are the result of positive thinking and having optimistic attitudes:

- Improved stress control and better general coping skills
- Better psychological health
- stronger resistance to infections such as the common cold
- Increased sense of well-being
- Improved longevity
- Lower depression
- Lesser risk of heart disease and related death

How do the scientists explain this strong correlation?

According to some research, people who think and see things positively are usually not severely affected by stress. Positive thinking helps them deal with stressful situations with less damage and they survive stressful events in life with a sense of more meaning in their lives.

Another theory is that positive thinkers usually live healthier lives in general; they are more active, eat a healthier diet and stay away from unhealthy habits.

There is a time when positive is just too positive

Scientists found that people can overdo positive thinking when a more realistic outlook would be more helpful. Positive thinking can make people blind to the reality of some situations so they tend to make inaccurate judgments and bad decisions.

Also, positive people always expect a positive outcome and the disappointment when things go wrong can be crushing and affect them in a very bad way.

That does not mean that it is better to be a pessimist. In the long run, positive thinking is more beneficial but a more realistic outlook is usually the best approach.

How to practice positive thinking

One strategy to improve your ability to see things in a more positive light is being aware of your thoughts and consciously switching from negative thoughts to positive ones when you notice that you are leaning in that way. Positive self-talk and gratitude awareness also help in being more positive.

The pros and cons of positive thinking

According to the studies on positive thinking, a positive outlook helps people have healthier and happier lives. It makes them healthier as they tend to exercise more, eat better and sleep enough.

On the flip side, positive thinking encourages unreasonable expectations which cause painful disappointment.

We can consciously change from negative to positive thinking

If you are determined to change from a negative to a positive outlook, try practicing mindfulness. It helps build self-awareness and consciousness of negative thoughts when they start dominating. Once being aware of them, you can take deliberate steps to move to more positive thinking. With practice, you are building a habit, and building better habits is one of the key tools to having a happier life.

Chapter 8

What comes first: success or happiness?

When reaching midlife, many women feel guilty for not achieving what we consider in our modern world success. That is normally equated with financial and material wealth. We feel like it is somehow our fault and that it is the main reason why we are not happy now. Let's examine just how big a part our material and financial success mean for our happiness.

The secret to happiness has been obsessing philosophers, poets, scientists, and the rest of us throughout history. We discussed in previous chapters the definition of happiness, what makes us happy and what does not. Success seems to be one of those things that do not make us happy.

On the contrary, the research shows that happiness brings success, not the other way around. How does that work? Don't we all spend our lives working hard in order to be more successful so that one day it can bring us happiness? Well, it appears that we should start by working on being happy first and then success would come.

However counter-intuitive this sounds, the research is solid and it tells us some very useful things.

We can agree on what contributes to success: intelligence, expertise in our field, social support and fitness. But, scientists believe that happiness is one of the crucial ingredients as well. Professor Lyubomirsky, who spent years researching happiness, says that "happy individuals are more likely than their less happy peers to have fulfilling marriages and relationships, high incomes, superior work performance, community involvement, robust health and even a long life."

Why do happy people earn more and get rich and successful more often than unhappy people?

Happiness makes people more productive. They are more content with their jobs, and when people like their jobs, they are good at it and consequently, they earn more than their colleagues. They are more confident and consequently make faster and better decisions. Happiness improves their problem-solving ability as well.

In addition, a sense of hopefulness and enthusiasm tends to reduce our risk of heart disease by half. This is explained by the fact that happy people engage in healthier behavior.

Happy people have more friends, and are more popular and loved

This is not surprising. Everyone loves hanging out with happy people. They are cheerful and positive and it seems like their optimism is contagious.

Happy people are more generous

Another reason happy people are liked is that they tend to be generous, with their time, attention, help, and money. They thrive when helping others and sharing what they have. This sharing is something we will return to later, it is one of the biggest secrets to happiness.

Happy people enjoy better relationships and marriages

It is almost impossible to be happy on your own. Being a part of a community, a group, a family or a relationship is a crucial ingredient for happiness. But it works the other way around too: happy people form stronger relationships and better marriages because of their need to share, empathy, and need to help.

Being conscious of the needs and feelings of those around us and offering to help when help is needed is a big part of who happy people are. Can we call it good Karma?

Happy people are healthier

Scientific evidence shows that happy people are mentally and physically healthier than unhappy people. They are more resilient to diseases, less prone to stress and generally lead healthier lives. The connection between stress and both mental and physical health has been well-researched. It is not difficult to understand that happy people, who are less sensitive to stress, tend to be more resistant to many diseases and more mentally stable.

People who are obsessed with working their entire lives in order to accumulate material wealth do not spend much time taking care of their health and well-being. They also sacrifice their social and family life and relationship with their children.

Happy people are more resilient and calmer

Happy people are not always happy. Life does not work like that. But when hardships and tragedies strike, they are able to cope better and bounce back faster. They take negative experiences as opportunities to grow and learn.

Happy people cope with tragedies better and help others to do the same. They are calmer in difficult situations and control their emotions better. Their positive mindset leads them to find the way out of any difficult situation and to find a solution out of any trouble.

Their strong social circle provides them with a powerful support system in their times of need and they are not hesitant to lean on that support.

Happy people deal with physical diseases better, by finding a way to laugh and joke while going through pain and therapy. This positive attitude is a strong boost to the immune system.

Lina's story

In her mid-40s, Lina was diagnosed with cancer. The diagnosis itself is enough to throw many people into depression. But she was not the type. Being a generally happy and positive person, she decided to do everything in her power to beat the odds. She went online and researched everything she could about her type of cancer. She found the best possible specialists near her. The doctors came up with a treatment plan and she started six weeks of a combination of chemotherapy and radiation therapy.

Despite it all, the main question that runs through the minds of all cancer patients is always, "Am I going to survive this?" Lina asked her doctor, a wise older man, what makes some people survive and others not when they have the same disease and the same treatment.

The doctor told her that he and the medicine can do their part, but much of what is needed is up to her. Some people have inner strength, determination, and a positive outlook that often beat even the worse odds. The doctor refused to call it a miracle. He called it 'the power of positivity.'

Happiness Formula

Don't laugh. The scientists actually came up with a happiness formula. They just cannot help it. Here it is: H=S+C+V. H is for happiness, S for set point (genetic factors), C for the person's circumstances, and V for actions under person's control.

Here is the problem. These elements do not contribute equally to our happiness. It appears that genetics take 50 percent, our life circumstances take 10 percent and only 40 percent of our happiness is under our real control.

The happiness in the formula is enduring happiness, not a temporary state that goes up and down. It is not the happiness that can be fixed by a trip to a spa or a trip to Hawaii.

Let's see what we can do with these elements of our happiness.

S: Set Range. This is happiness that depends on our genetic profile. It seems that about half of our happiness potential is already predetermined by our genes. It means that some of us are by nature positive and we naturally gravitate toward happiness. Some people are naturally surly and sullen and we just accept it as their nature. Most of us are somewhere in between.

What does this mean? It means that whatever happens in our life, we tend to gravitate toward our natural happiness level. Naturally happy people can survive the worst tragedies, become crippled and in a short time bounce back and return to their happy selves. Naturally unhappy people can win a lottery and will be ecstatic for a while but soon after they will return to their surliness.

We cannot do much about this part of the formula but we have two more elements to work with and those we can influence.

C: Circumstances. Here are some suggestions on how to improve your circumstances in order to improve this element of your happiness:

- If your circumstance is to live in an impoverished country or in a dictatorship, get out and move to a country where freedom and democracy are a part of everyone's circumstances.
- Get into a steady relationship or get married
- Stay out of negative events and avoid negative emotions
- Build a strong social network
- Stay healthy
- Get as much education as possible.
- Improve your economic situation

Many of these conditions are impossible or hard to change, but people keep trying. Refugees and immigrants are trying every day at great costs. No wonder these hard-to-change elements contribute only ten percent to our happiness.

V: Voluntary Variables. This is the element we can work with and which contributes 40 percent to our happiness. But, you will be surprised to see the conditions necessary to change this variable:

- You have to think positively about your past (with satisfaction, fulfillment, contentment, serenity, and pride)
- You have to think positively about the future (with optimism, faith, hope, and trust)
- You have to have positive emotions about your present (feel joy, calm, pleasure, and flow)

So, to be happier, you have to change your feelings and the way you think about your past, present and future. That is all? It is not as easy as it looks.

The past

The way you feel about your past can color your present and your future. Your disappointments, anger, resentment and self-pity can severely affect your present happiness. On the other side, if you feel fulfilled, content, proud, and serene about your past, it makes a big impact on how happy you feel now.

Sounds simple? Yes, and if you dig into your personal feelings about your past, you will realize just how right it is.

The good thing is that we can affect how we feel about the past. Martin Seligman, the father of Positive Psychology, suggests three strategies:

- **Stop believing that your past decides your future.** It makes you passive and fatalistic. Tell yourself that you cannot change the past but your present is in your hands and under your control, and so is your happiness. Learn from the past but leave it in the past.

- **Be grateful for everything good in your past.** Your gratitude for the past—good things, events, and experiences—focuses on the good that happened. Try to remember all the good things by writing them down. They are all part of who you are now.

- **Forgive bad things from the past.** Forgiving the wrongs from your past removes their power over you and prevents bitterness that can color your life. Holding on to a grudge, resentment, anger, or hate is like holding the poison that slowly leaks and is affecting your present happiness.

The future

How you feel about your future—hopeful, optimistic, trustful, anxious, afraid, or horrified—is mostly formed by how you see and interpret your world.

If you believe that you are going to fail that next week's exam, you will be miserable, but if you are feeling good about how well-prepared you are and how successful you will be, you will be happy long before it happens.

Since it appears that it is all in our heads, that is where we have to fight it. Recognize and discard negative, pessimistic thoughts. Realize that it is a matter of perspective. It is how your mind interprets the events, not the events themselves.

The present – pleasure vs. gratification

To feel better about your present, you need to learn the difference between pleasure and gratification.

Pleasures are derived through our senses and emotions: thrills, ecstasy, exuberance, orgasm, delight, mirth, and comfort. Pleasures are generally temporary and seldom involve any thinking. Some pleasant activities are watching TV, listening to music, eating chocolate, or drinking wine.

Gratifications are activities that do not involve emotions but involve us entirely. We get absorbed in them and stop being self-conscious. It happens when our skills are equal to the challenge. We engage all our strengths and are aware of them. It feels like we are 'in the flow" and time has stopped.

Some of the examples are playing a sport we love, helping others, climbing a mountain, having an interesting conversation, dancing, or reading a really good book.

The gratifications tend to last longer than the pleasures and involve a lot of thinking,

When your gratifications are bigger and more numerous than your pleasures, you can achieve lasting happiness. Chasing pleasures is not the way to be truly happy, regardless of how pleasant it feels at the moment.

How to increase gratifications?

Start by asking yourself what is it you are doing when you feel that you are 'in the flow.' What it is that you want to keep doing and do not want to stop. In Positive Psychology, these activities are called our signature strengths.

Signature strengths are character strengths that are the essence of who we are. Some examples are creativity, ingenuity, curiosity, exploration, critical thinking, openness to experiences, open-mindedness, love of learning, or learning new skills.

For lasting happiness, try to discover your signature strengths. You might not even be aware of them. When you figure them out, try to use them whenever you can. They will hugely increase your lasting satisfaction with life and your happiness.

Discover your signature strengths

Signature strengths are character strengths that are essential to who we really are. We do not always know our essential strengths. To find out which of your strengths are the most important of all and which define you, you have to ask yourself some important questions:

- What strengths or personality characteristics define you as a person?
- Is that strength energizing?
- Is it used easily?
- Is it used in any setting?

The research shows that two-thirds of people are not completely aware of their signature or most important strengths, at least not to the extent to be using them with any meaning. This is important as it shows that we often do not use the character features that are the most important for the kind of person we are. They matter to us and to our sense of identity.

Three main features of our character strengths – the three Es

- **Essential**: that is the strength that is essential to your personality, to who you really are;
- **Effortless**: when you are using that strength it feels effortless and natural;
- **Energizing**: using your signature strength makes you feel uplifted, in balance, happy, and ready for anything.

The key is to spot and recognize your strengths as signature strengths and use them to their full potential.

How to spot our signature strengths?

We know our strengths, but often do not realize just how crucial they are to who we are. Here are a few examples of people using their signature strengths without being aware of them:

After taking VIA Institute of Character test about character strengths, Eva found out to her surprise that curiosity is her main, number one strength of character. After thinking about it, she realized just how true it is. She always asks hundreds of questions, is interested in just about everything, and loves to travel and discover new places.

This characteristic made Eva connect with people very easily; asking questions to total strangers on the bus, chatting with neighbors, and always interested in everything they have to say. This is not only the way she connected to people but what made her very much liked by people and even by potential employers. And her curiosity made her always happy and cheerful.

For Sue, surprising signature strength was prudence. Prudence, linked to 'being a prude' and boring, has a bad rap. But, prudence means being cautious and cautiously wise, choosing things carefully, and thinking before speaking.

In Sue's life, her signature strength made her careful and not take too many risks. She was blaming herself for not living her life to the fullest. She tended to hold back in new situations. But, when looking back at her life, Sue realized that her prudence served her very well indeed. It made her a very successful project manager, known for being goal-oriented, well-organized, and conscientious. All those things that come to her easily and naturally.

So, instead of feeling guilty for not living a full life because of her prudence, Sue realized that her life was full and the risks she did take were just much more carefully thought through before taking action. That realization made her appreciate herself and her accomplishments much more than before.

Can you recognize your signature strengths? Have a look at the list of the VIA Classification of Character Strengths list and identify strengths that best describe who you are deep down. Look for the strengths that are for you **essential**, **effortless,** and **energizing.**

VIA CLASSIFICATION OF CHARACTER STRENGTHS

The Virtue of Wisdom

- Creativity: Original; adaptive; ingenuity
- Curiosity: Interest; novelty-seeking; exploration; openness to experience
- Judgment: Critical thinking; thinking things through; open-minded
- Love of Learning: Mastering new skills & topics; systematically adding to knowledge
- Perspective: Wisdom; providing wise counsel; taking the big picture view

The Virtue of Courage

- Bravery: Valor; not shrinking from fear; speaking up for what's right
- Perseverance: Persistence; industry; finishing what one starts
- Honesty: Authenticity; integrity
- Zest: Vitality; enthusiasm; vigor; energy; feeling alive and activated

The Virtue of Humanity

- Love: Both loving and being loved; valuing close relations with others
- Kindness: Generosity; nurturance; care; compassion; altruism; "niceness"
- Social Intelligence: Aware of the motives/feelings of oneself & others

The Virtue of Justice

- Teamwork: Citizenship; social responsibility; loyalty
- Fairness: Just; not letting feelings bias decisions about others
- Leadership: Organizing group activities; encouraging a group to get things done

The Virtue of Temperance

- Forgiveness: Mercy; accepting others' shortcomings; giving people a second chance
- Humility: Modesty; letting one's accomplishments speak for themselves
- Prudence: Careful; cautious; not taking undue risks
- Self-Regulation: Self-control; disciplined; managing impulses & emotions

The Virtue of Transcendence

- Appreciation of Beauty and Excellence: Awe; wonder; elevation
- Gratitude: Thankful for the good; expressing thanks; feeling blessed
- Hope: Optimism; future-mindedness; future orientation
- Humor: Playfulness; bringing smiles to others; lighthearted
- Spirituality: Religiousness; faith; purpose; meaning

Source: VIA Institute of Character

You can take the VIA Survey to get your personalized Top 5 Report and check just how accurate your own identification of your strengths was. There is a cost involved, though.

You might find that many of the listed characteristics describe you pretty well. Try to find the five that are the most important. Always think about things that come to you easily and which you could always do with great pleasure.

But this is not the end of discussing your signature strengths. Look at each of them and try to see whether you are using them to your full potential. Are you doing them often enough? Each of them can and should be your guiding force in life, the strengths that should be used to fulfill your true potential.

Be happy to be successful

OK, we can understand now that it is more useful to start happy and become successful because our happiness is an important prerequisite for success. Yes, but how? It is not like we did not want to start happy so we can become successful. If we knew how, we would not be discussing all this.

Lasting happiness is an inner characteristic of people who learned that there are some things that are necessary for happiness. Here are some of them:

Be grateful to those who were good to you

Try writing letters to people you are grateful to, even if you do not plan on sending them. Just acknowledging your gratitude to those who were good to you will fill you with happiness that will last for weeks.

Be always optimistic

For whatever is happening or you plan on doing, start by visualizing a positive outcome. It will not only increase the chance of a positive outcome but will make you happy long before the event.

Count all your blessings

Writing about three good things that happened to you each week will lift your spirit and make you feel lighter and happier.

Use your strengths

Identify your signature strengths and make an effort to use them more often and in new ways. You will be surprised how good it will make you feel.

Be kind to others

Be always kind to people, even total strangers. It will give you a feeling of constant well-being.

Hope vs. Optimism

We discussed in many chapters the importance of being optimistic and having a positive attitude in order to be happier. The problem is that we are often confusing optimism with hope.

According to the Cambridge Dictionary, **hope** is "something good that you want to happen in the future, or a confident feeling about what will happen in the future." **Optimism** is defined as "the quality of being full of hope and emphasizing the good parts of a situation or a belief that something good will happen."

It means that hope is about someone's **beliefs** about themselves and what they plan to do in order to reach their goals. Beliefs are not necessarily accurate. Hope is a person's lasting but not permanent state of mind, linked to a certain event, and it depends on the situation.

On the other side, optimism is about someone's nature, about being a "glass-half-full" kind of person. We believe that optimists are people who were born optimistic. The scientists do not quite agree with that.

Optimism describes a person's character trait that does not depend on any event or outside situation. A person expects that good things will happen in the future and bad, undesired things will not.

Scientists such as Martin Seligman, the *Father of Positive Psychology*, believe that being an optimist can be learned and is not something we are born with. This is very good news as it means that we can teach ourselves to be more optimistic, one of the necessary conditions for happiness.

In several studies, scientists investigated the difference between states that are about the future: optimism, hope, wish, want, desire, and joy. Their conclusion is that hoping is closest to wishing but not the same. It is different from optimism because it is an emotion.

Hope represents a more important and less likely result and it offers much less control. Hope means personal investment in a situation in which chances are poor. Both hope and optimism are considered positive states and are the sign of good psychological health.

Chapter 9

Joy is an inside-outside job

Joy vs. happiness

Now that we have trashed happiness in all its shapes, forms and incarnations, we have one more job to do; to find out if it is actually happiness we are seeking, or is it joy.

Some people use the two words interchangeably, but there is a profound difference between the two. They are so different that you can actually choose one or another. And maybe you can choose both.

It of course depends on the definition of happiness you subscribe to, but generally, happiness is an emotion that you experience while it is happening to you, and it depends on different external factors. You desire happiness and pursue it, but you cannot choose happiness consciously.

On the other hand, joy is a choice, something you make deliberately and purposefully. Joy is your unused potential, always there, inside you. It is the attitude towards life chosen by your spirit and your heart. That is the reason you can feel joy even while going through the toughest times.

It is not necessary to smile to show that you experience joy. You can experience joy while feeling a range of other emotions such as anger, sadness, or shame. You cannot possibly be happy while experiencing those feelings.

Happiness usually disappears when you are going through difficult times, but joy persists. It is rooted deeply in your spirit. It provides you with peace and serenity in your life. We pursue happiness but ultimately choose joy.

Joy is more consistent than happiness, which we accepted is not permanent. We cultivate joy internally.

The conditions for experiencing joy

You can experience joy only when you accept and make peace with who you truly are. Happiness is usually triggered externally and it depends on other people, places, thoughts, things, and events.

Since joy is more permanent, less transitory and not linked to outside circumstances, having joy in life is better than just having happiness.

One way to look at the difference between happiness and joy is that you want happiness for yourself but joy is what you feel when you want happiness for others. You feel joy when you care for other people, when you are thankful or when you have spiritual experiences.

Joy often requires self-sacrifice, but provides you with lasting inner peace and contentment.

Here are some significant differences between happiness and joy that can help you decide which one is right for you. There is no wrong choice, seeking each of them will make your life better, but it will be a different kind of life.

1. Joy is lasting but happiness is temporary.

Having a baby is a source of constant joy that lasts a lifetime. In comparison, winning a lottery provides a feeling of happiness that lasts for a while, but soon it will be just a memory.

2. Joy means happiness for others, happiness is about ourselves.

When you are being selfless, you think about the good of others and not about your own feelings. This is often challenging but it brings a lot of joy and provides meaning and purpose to your life.

Being happy is fun but it does not have a meaning besides making us content. Good food makes you happy but it is not a meaningful act. When you prepare the meal yourself, it brings you the pleasure of good food but also of feeding your family or friends.

3. Joy is often deeply spiritual, while happiness has little depth.

Enjoying a piece of chocolate gives you great pleasure for a brief time. Taking care of an animal brings you joy, because of the bond you are creating between you, but also because of caring for another life.

4. Joy has a meaning while happiness just feels good.

Experiencing joy is profound and often memorable. Seeing your child smile for the first time or watching your mother laugh bring lasting memories that bring you joy every time you think of them. Buying a new pair of shoes is very nice but the good feeling lasts only a short time.

5. Joy is a choice and happiness is something people chase.

When you are looking for a job that you do not like but which brings a great salary, you believe that it will bring you happiness. You soon realize that you were wrong and that the salary is not enough. When you choose a job that is not well-paid but is meaningful or that you enjoy and are good at, that job will bring you lasting joy.

6. Joy often involves hardships, while happiness is usually easier to have.

Working in a refugee camp is very hard and often heartbreaking, but it brings you great joy when you see the faces of people whose lives you are making better. Going to a big sale at the department store makes you happy because of all the big bargains you will enjoy buying things, but the happiness will last a short time, usually until you realize that you really did not need those clothes and that you should have saved the money.

7. Joy is transformative but happiness can hold you back.

Experiencing joy can be profound and transformative. When you spend an hour on the computer chatting with a person who was thinking about suicide and needed someone to talk to, that experience can profoundly transform you and bring you joy by helping a human being in crisis.

When you spend an hour browsing through meaningless comments on your Facebook, you will have fun while it lasts but when you are done, you will realize that you have just wasted an hour of your time that you could have spent studying or helping kids with their homework.

8. Joy truly connects people, while connections that bring happiness are often short lasting and shallow.

Meeting a new friend at the mountain climbing club might mean a lifetime friendship between two people who share the same interest and joy. Meeting people in a bar, where it is too noisy for a conversation and where getting drunk is the main goal is a short-lasting pleasure.

9. Joy is less common than happiness, and is much stronger.

Joy is not common because it requires that you know and accept yourself and are willing to undergo hardship to achieve it. For that reason, many people do not want it. For them, the pleasure of happiness is good enough. Happiness is easier and requires less effort, so people seek it even when they know that it is not long-lasting.

10. Joy is difficult to define, happiness is not.

Not many people know what joy really is but everyone can easily describe happiness. A profound experience and feeling that makes us fulfilled, content and in balance is difficult to describe. Happiness is a familiar feeling and most people experience it from time to time and can easier describe it.

11. Joy lasts through hardship, happiness does not.

Joy survives difficult situations but happiness disappears when things get hard. You can feel joy even when you are experiencing loss or pain, but you cannot feel happy in such circumstances.

Finding true joy

Now that you understand better the difference between joy and happiness, you might feel that you are ready for this deeper, more meaningful feeling of well-being. Once you realize just how profound a difference it can make to the quality of your life, you will start wondering how you can go about achieving it.

Here are just a few ways:

Volunteer: There is an endless number of ways you can give your time, your skills and your compassion to those in need. You can volunteer in your church, in the local soup kitchen, you can spend a year volunteering in some developing country, or you can teach your neighbor's kid how to play piano. Volunteering is when you offer a shoulder to someone going through a tough time to cry on, help an old lady cross the street, or buy groceries for your home-bound neighbor. Just open your heart and accept that you have enough love in you to share it with those around you.

You will do your best when you offer help doing a job you love and enjoy. When you use your signature character skills, you share the best of yourself, and you are filled with joy at the same time.

Keep a journal: When you write down about the events in your day, you have a better understanding of your motivations and what makes you tick. You can go back to previous days, weeks and years and piece together how your joy stays constant in your life. Even when things are tough, and when you are in pain, you have the knowledge and clarity of purpose and meaning in your life.

Your journal will also help you see when you make wrong decisions or hurt someone inadvertently. When you lose your focus and doubt yourself. You can see the side of yourself you do not like and work on it.

Accept yourself for who you are: When you are true to yourself, you surround yourself with people who like you exactly the way you are. They boost your confidence and share your love.

Once you accept yourself completely, you can fulfill your dreams and find your purpose. You can devote yourself to the job your love. Most importantly, nothing other people say or do to hurt you can touch you. You can allow yourself to be eccentric and whimsical and try new things and explore new horizons.

Be creative: allow yourself to enjoy a hobby that fulfills you on a different level, which allows you to dig deep down into your personality that is not always obvious. Enjoy the beauty of art for the sake of beauty.

Meet people: Find time for people you love or admire. Talk to them about your day, discuss current events or just laugh together about life's silliness. Let people talk to you and listen to them with focus, even when you do not agree with them. Listen to people you admire and learn what they have to teach you.

Meet new people and listen to different ideas and perspectives. Join clubs where people do things you love doing. That is the best way to meet people who can become great friends or even someone you can love.

Meditate: In your busy life, you have to find time to take a break. Meditation will allow you to let your mind stop churning and unwind. It allows your body and mind to regain balance and peace.

Meditation is not some esoteric skill you have to go to Tibet to learn. All it means is to stop thinking and breathe.

How to meditate

You can find a video or join a nearby club to learn how to meditate, but it is not that difficult to learn once you demystify it and learn what it really means. It can be done anywhere and at any time.

1. Sit or lay down, whatever makes you most comfortable. Close your eyes.

2. Take several deep breaths. Breathe in through the nose and out through the mouth. Focus on your breathing and follow the path of air through your body.

3. Your thoughts will intrude. Let them, acknowledge them and let them go.

4. Start thinking about your body. Start with the head, then your neck, shoulders, arms, hands, chest, stomach, back and legs, until you reach the toes.

5. As you become aware of each part of the body, try to release the tension in each of them. Consciously relax them while you are breathing. Try relaxing each muscle by first squeezing it to become aware of it.

6. Focus on breathing again. When you are completely relaxed, slowly open your eyes.

7. Before moving, be aware of how you are feeling and how it compares with the way you felt before the meditation.

Each session can last as short or as long as you need. You can have a quick session before an important meeting or after a stressful encounter. Accept meditation as a part of your life that is meant to help you live better and healthier.

Meditation does not require a special position, special clothes, or a special place, but if you enjoy creating a little ritual out of it, go for it. Just breathe and relax. With practice, you will find that you can completely detach from your surroundings.

How to practice forgiveness

There are some parts of creating a more meaningful and fulfilled life that are really hard. Forgiveness is one of them. But however painful it is, it is necessary for your peace of mind.

Life can deal us some really hard hits and nobody is immune to them. It is difficult to even imagine forgiving someone who hurt you or someone you love, betrayed you, abandoned you or lied to you. When you are a victim of a crime or are being bullied, all you can think about is pain, hurt, or revenge.

But holding to that pain and hurt is preventing you from going on with your life and enjoying normal relationships. The only way to regain balance and joy in your life is through forgiveness.

Forgiveness heals even the deepest wounds but is very hard to achieve. Some people believe that they never could.

Here are some basic steps you can try to adapt to your situation and your life. Give them time to work and accept that the effort and work that is required are worthwhile and necessary.

What forgiveness is and why it is important

Forgiveness is based on your inner goodness. It is about showing mercy to people who have hurt us, even if you believe that they don't "deserve" it. It does not mean finding an excuse or justification for that person's actions. It has nothing to do with pretending that it didn't happen.

There is no recipe or quick formula you can use. Forgiveness is a long process with various necessary steps that do not follow the same order for each person.

Working through all steps towards forgiveness will help you boost your self-esteem and fortify your inner strength and a sense of safety. It can show how wrong the lies we tell ourselves when we are deeply hurt are, such as "I am unworthy," or "I am completely defeated."

Forgiveness has the power to heal us and let us go on with our life with purpose and meaning. When forgiving, you are the main beneficiary, not the person you are forgiving.

Research shows that forgiving someone offers a powerful psychological benefit to the person offering forgiveness. It can lower depression, reduce anxiety and unhealthy anger, and many symptoms of PTSD.

We don't forgive just to help ourselves. Forgiveness leads to psychological healing, but it is not about you or for you. It is something you do for another person because you know that in the long run, it is the best response to a difficult situation.

Learn 'forgiveness fitness'

Just like exercise, forgiveness requires practice and it is best to start slowly. You need to incorporate forgiveness 'practice.'

Start by committing yourself to never harming anyone. It means making a conscious effort not to talk bad things about the person that hurt you. You do not need to say good things either, just stop yourself from saying bad things. That will "feed" your forgiving side.

Practice recognizing that each person is special and irreplaceable. Whether you reach this recognition through your religion, your humanist philosophy, or your belief in evolution, it is important to nurture this mindset of recognizing the value of our common humanity. That makes it harder to discount a person who has hurt you as valueless.

The power of love

Another way to practice forgiveness is to show love in some small way to the random people you meet during the day. Smile to the mailman, give a compliment to the grocery store cashier, or listen to a neighbor's child. This builds your 'love muscle' and the skill of showing compassion to everyone.

Try showing compassion and forgiveness to people that hurt you or who are unkind to you, just to practice. Hold your tongue when you want to lash out when someone insults you or is being rude.

Get rid of pride

Pride and a sense of power might make you feel entitled or inflate your sense of importance, weakening your efforts to practice forgiveness. They can make you hold on to your resentment and a feeling of being a victim. Catch yourself when behaving like this and switch to forgiveness and mercy.

If you need some help with this, you can read some true stories at the <u>International Forgiveness Institute</u>.

Deal with your inner pain

It is necessary to understand who has hurt you in your life and how. This seems obvious, but it is not. Some actions that hurt you are not unjust. When your partner is being rude or your child is being a brat, it hurts but you do not have to forgive them.

When you look back to people in your life who hurt you in various ways, you will find that the hurt comes in different shapes. Sometimes you were not given love or were physically punished. You need to acknowledge all these pains because they all add up to your inner pain. That will allow you to understand who should be forgiven, and that can be the place to start from.

Emotional pain comes in many forms: anxiety, anger, depression, lack of trust, low self-esteem, self-loathing, a negative worldview, or a lack of confidence to be able to change. Forgiveness heals all these hurts. Identify the kind of pain you suffer from and acknowledge it. The more you have been hurt, the more important it is to forgive so that you can heal.

Do not hesitate to seek help from a therapist if you cannot do the accounting for all your pains on your own. Sometimes a good friend can help, as long as you feel supported and safe when doing it.

Use empathy for nurturing a forgiving mind

The research shows that there is a link between imagining forgiveness and the brain's neural circuit activity responsible for empathy. It means that empathy is linked to forgiveness. Feeling empathy is a crucial step in the forgiveness process.

If you are willing to look into the details of the life of the person who hurt you, you will see the wounds that person carries, triggering empathy for that person. Start by imagining him as a child, in need of support and love. Did he get enough of it from his parents?

Research shows that a child who does not receive enough love and attention from his caregivers will be unable to develop strong attachments, and as a consequence will not be able to trust. That can create a cycle of conflict and loneliness that will affect that person's entire life.

Once you start seeing the suffering the person who hurt you has endured, you can see the common human frailties you share. You will be able to accept that regardless of the suffering that person has caused you, he does not deserve suffering, just like you do not, and deserves your forgiveness.

Find meaning in the suffering

You do not have to be a Buddhist to understand this. It helps to endure suffering if you can find that it means something. Without it, it is easy to feel the loss of a purpose, hopelessness and desperation and the feeling that life itself has no meaning. The answer is in finding the meaning in what we have endured, the way our suffering has changed us for the better.

Realizing that their suffering has made them more resilient and more courageous, some people are able to keep developing short and long-term life goals because they can see how suffering has changed their perspective, their priorities in life, and understanding of what really matters.

Finding meaning does not necessarily make pain less, but it makes the best of it. It helps to believe that everything happens for a reason. Nevertheless, you need to recognize that what happened to you was unjust so that your forgiveness has proper meaning.

There are many ways of finding meaning in suffering. It can be by sharing your experience with others and helping them learn how to forgive. Or you can just try to learn to be more loving and to share your love with others.

Chapter 10

Now it's your turn

So here we are. You have gone through all the chapters, gotten all the tools and weapons, and are now ready to embark on the adventure of transformation and better and more meaningful life. But before that, let's get one thing clear:

You are fine just the way you are. There is nothing wrong with you. There is nothing wrong in not wanting to change your life or disrupt everything you know about. You can, but you do not have to.

Reaching midlife brings with it many physical and hormonal changes and the fact that it means half of our life is over makes us contemplate mortality and wonder about what it is all about. It is normal, almost everyone goes through it.

We have discussed some of the ways you can go through this process so it does not turn into a crisis. If you are in control of it, it is not a crisis. Whether you want to make changes to the life you have now and make that future life better and more meaningful, it is in your hands. You are in control.

To make that decision to change your life drastically, just a little bit or not at all, is not easy. You have gotten the tools through this book, but how are you going to use them for the best is a decision you have to make. Maybe you should get just a little bit of help. Let's recap what we have discussed so far about different aspects of happiness to see where you stand on them.

Success

You now understand that success does not necessarily mean a powerful career and lot of money. You also understand how unrealistic expectations can sabotage your happiness. So, ask yourself; what do you really want to succeed in? You do not like your job but is finding a new one in your 50s really unrealistic? You can make your job more interesting by learning more about it, research new discoveries, learn to do it the best way you can. Take courses online. Look for a different job in your company that is more interesting to you.

If you want to change your job and your circumstances allow it, go for it, but before you decide what to do, evaluate your strengths and skills. What you are good at and what you can offer. Once you have clear idea what kind of job you want, go for it, apply, look for a head-hunter or ask friends for help.

If you have been a housewife your whole life and did not have a career, it does not mean that you did not have a job. You raised the kids, the most important job of all. You can give more time to your hobbies. Or take courses online to learn new things. Go volunteer. All that will give you the feeling of success.

Ask yourself if the job you have has a meaning, if it gives you a satisfaction that you are doing something that makes life better for others in some way. Any job can have more meaning if you want it to.

Empowerment

While going through previous chapters, you have learned the tricks and tips to boost your self-esteem and resilience, to discover your key strengths and to conquer your fears. All those tools make you capable of making the changes you want, but you have to decide what changes you really want to make. What is it that you want? What would really make you happy?

This is true empowerment: to have the power over your life and the decisions you make. You decide whether you want to completely change your life, or you are really fine with what you have, just want to shake it up a bit. It takes courage and a really empowered woman to say: I did all this, and I am grateful for what I have achieved. It is not perfect, but it is a good life. I have a great loving family, plenty of good friends, a job that is boring but pays the bills and pays for the kids' education. I have my hobbies to do things I really love. I spend time volunteering at the school for blind children, making their lives better.

That is a picture of a good life, if that is how you see it. If that gives you happiness, that is what happiness is for you. And accepting this does not mean giving up dreams and should not make you feel guilty. In fact, it should make you feel relieved because you are now clear about what you want and what is truly important to you.

It is possible that your feeling of empowerment allows you to drastically change your life. Empowerment and the right circumstances. You do not have any family that depends on you and your family and friends are encouraging you to go after your dreams. You are aware that the big changes, such as moving to another country, mean not having the support of your friends and family and that you will be often very much alone. You will probably not have the support of the infrastructure, health care and financial system you are used to. Are you prepared for all that? If you have done enough research and are prepared to embark on a huge adventure without a parachute, then go for it. You will find that you are not alone in it.

There are entire communities of expats in various countries full of people who cut the ties with their previous lives and started a completely new life. Lawyers became dive masters, teachers started volunteering in small local schools, and many highly educated people decided to spend the rest of their lives volunteering, reading, writing, walking, hiking, hanging out with similar people. And having the life of their dreams.

It often means living on much less money that you are used to. Living in a one-room beach shack, having to travel by boat to the nearest doctor or having to subsist on the local produce and having very little access to the little luxuries such as good wine or organic strawberries. But the sense of freedom is indescribable.

Happiness and joy

Another thing you have to decide, and being empowered and aware of your true self, have the knowledge and insight for, is what kind of happiness you want. The term 'joy' might make you uncomfortable because it sounds vaguely New Age-ish, but all it really means is a different word for happiness that is turned outside, towards others.

So, do you want to work on happiness you know more about, and making everything in your life better, or are you willing to give up some of the comforts and pleasures of that kind of happiness to go after more lasting, and in the long run, more fulfilling kind of happiness? Because joy means devoting your life to making your life have more meaning by making others happier, even if it means sacrificing your own happiness.

If you are truly strong and determined, you might be able to have both. Because having your life full of meaning and purpose does not mean living in a monastery or temple but making sure that your life is making someone's life better, even if it is one person only. By giving your free time to teach underprivileged children, you are making a difference in those kids' lives. By working pro bono as a lawyer for the refugees is ensuring that their rights are respected.

And sometimes, happiness and joy come in a completely unexpected direction. It is not rare to meet mothers who spent their whole lives raising their children to be good human beings and devoted their lives to their well-being. Or daughters who spent years taking care of their sick parents, never resenting it and feeling fulfilled and happy.

We all come in different shapes, forms, desires, and dreams. We need and want different things. But as long as we are free and empowered to decide how to live our lives and to make decisions about our lives, we can achieve happiness.

Now it's your turn. You know who you are and what you can and cannot do. You accept yourself for who you truly are and you are proud of yourself. You know how to respect what you have and what is really important to you. You know that life is precious and short and that happiness is not a distant goal but that it is in here and now. And however much life is left, you plan on living it every day filled with happiness and purpose. Have a safe trip, be adventurous but risk carefully, enjoy your travels but remember to help others on your way.

Thank you

Thank you for taking the time to read this book. I hope that you had fun reading it, recognized yourself in it, had a few 'aha!' moments and at least a chuckle or two. I hope you can use the book to guide you through the stormy waters of middle age and show you the way out to a more fulfilled and happier second part of your life. If you liked the book and found it useful, please take a few minutes to leave a review HERE. It would be appreciated by the author but hopefully also by other women who need a bit of help with finding happiness.

References

Barton, J. & Pretty, J. (2010). *What is the best dose of nature and green exercise for improving mental health? A multi-study analysis.* Environmental Science and Technology. https://www.ncbi.nlm.nih.gov/pubmed/20337470

Blanchflower, David G. (2021). *Is happiness U-shaped everywhere? Age and subjective well-being in 145 countries.* Journal of Popular Economics. https://pubmed.ncbi.nlm.nih.gov/32929308/

Boehm, J. K., Peterson, C., Kivimaki, M., & Kubzansky, L. D. (2011). *Heart health when life is satisfying: evidence from the Whitehall II cohort study.* https://www.ncbi.nlm.nih.gov/pubmed/21727096

Brockis, J. (2019). *Why Happiness at Work Matters.* https://www.drjennybrockis.com/2019/1/24/happiness-work-matters/

Campos, D., Cebolla, A., Quero, S., Breton-Lopez, J., Botella, C., Soler, J., Garcia-Campayo, J., Demarzo, M., & Banos, R. M. (2016). *Meditation and happiness: Mindfulness and self-compassion may mediate the meditation–happiness relationship.* https://www.sciencedirect.com/science/article/pii/S0191886915005450

Cook, Claire. (2015). *Shine On: How to Grow Awesome Instead of Old.* Marshbury Beach Books.

Crossett, Sharon. *Feeling Lost in Your 40s*. Life coaching for women. https://www.lifecoachingforwomen.co.uk/news/feeling-lost-in-your-40s

Enright, Robert. (2015). *Eight Keys to Forgiveness*. Greater good magazine. https://greatergood.berkeley.edu/article/item/eight_keys_to_forgiveness

Kubzansky, Laura D. Thurston, Revecca C. (2007). *Emotional Vitality and Incident Coronary Heart Disease Benefits of Healthy Psychological Functioning*. Archives of General Psychiatry. https://jamanetwork.com/journals/jamapsychiatry/fullarticle/482515

Lyubomirsky, Sonja. (2008). *The How of Happiness*. Pinguin Books.

Niemiec, Ryan. (2015). *What do we know about signature strengths?* Positive Psychology News. https://positivepsychologynews.com/news/ryan-niemiec/2015042831514

Paganini-Hill, Annlia, Kawas, Claudia H. and Corrada, María M. (2018). *Positive Mental Attitude Associated with Lower 35-Year Mortality: The Leisure World Cohort Study*. Journal of Ageing Research. https://www.hindawi.com/journals/jar/2018/2126368/

Radmall, Andre. (2021). *Get Unstuck, Change the Script, Change your Life*. Rethink Press

Rockwell, Leah. (2021). *Midlife Crisis in Women: Signs, Causes, & How to Cope. Choosing Therapy*. Choosing Therapy. **https://www.choosingtherapy.com/midlife-crisis-women/**

Sandberg, Sharyl and Grant, Adam. (2017). *Option B: Facing Adversity, Building Resilience, and Finding Joy*. Knofp.

Sarkar, S.N. and Mishra, N.N. (1977). *A Study of Need for Achievement and Risk-Taking in Government Employees and Self-Employed Entrepreneurs.* Indian Anthropological Association. Vol. 7, No. 2 pp. 139-144. https://www.jstor.org/stable/41919322

Schutte, N. S., & Malouff, J. M. (2021). Using signature strengths to increase happiness at work. In J. Marques (Ed.), *The Routledge companion to happiness at work (pp. 13–22). Routledge/Taylor & Francis Group.* https://doi.org/10.4324/9780429294426-2

Shilling, Deb. (2015). You're Turning 40-Embracing Both Physical and Emotional Changes at this Milestone Birthday. Mankato Clinic. https://www.mankatoclinic.com/youre-turning-40?fbclid=IwAR27pPdACgxubRrwVuLbaowpsLaifymEqHwnmPyytFn0_ljlpORWwU8p8ss

Uliaszek, A.A., Rashid, T. & Zarowsky, Z. (2021). The role of signature strengths in treatment outcome: Initial results from a large and diverse university sample. Journal of Contemporary Psychotherapy. https://doi.org/10.1007/s10879-021-09523-6

Warren, M.A., Sekhon,T., & Waldrop, R. J. (2022). Highlighting strengths in response to discrimination: Developing and testing an allyship positive psychology intervention. International Journal of Wellbeing. https://doi.org/10.5502/ijw.v12i1.1751

Why Midlife Crises Are Different for Women and 6 ways to overcome them. Cleveland Clinic. https://health.clevelandclinic.org/why-midlife-crises-are-different-for-women/

Women's Health. (2020). *Why Midlife Crises Are Different for Women*

World Happiness Report (2022). https://worldhappiness.report/